Mom's Health Matters

Mom's Health Matters

PRACTICAL ANSWERS TO YOUR TOP HEALTH CONCERNS

Carrie Carter, M.D.

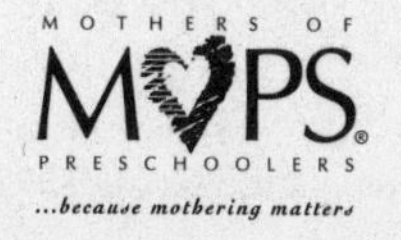

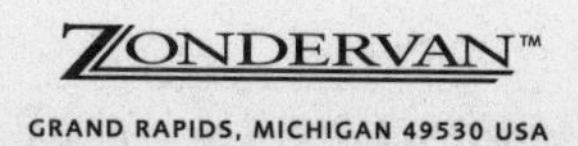

GRAND RAPIDS, MICHIGAN 49530 USA

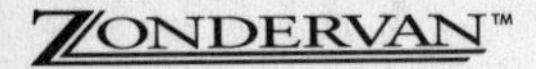

Mom's Health Matters

Requests for information should be addressed to:
Zondervan, *Grand Rapids, Michigan 49530*

Library of Congress Cataloging-in-Publication Data

Carter, Carrie, MD.
Mom's health matters : practical answers to your top health concerns / Carrie Carter.
p. cm.
Includes bibliographical references.
ISBN 0-310-24743-8
1. Mother's—Health and hygiene I. Title.
RA778.C2174 2003
613'.04244—dc21

2003012402

The website addresses recommended throughout this book are offered as a resource to you. These websites are not intended in any way to be or imply an endorsement on the part of Zondervan, nor do we vouch for their content for the life of this book.

Quote on pages 33–34 are taken from *Real Moms: Exploding the Myths of Motherhood* by Elisa Morgan and Carol Kuykendall. Used by permission of Zondervan.

Published in association with the literary agency of Alive Communications, Inc., 7680 Goddard Street, Suite 200, Colorado Springs, CO 80920.

Interior design by Nancy Wilson

Printed in the United States of America

03 04 05 06 07 08 09 /❖ DC/ 10 9 8 7 6 5 4 3 2

To the moms I've known in my medical practice.
Thank you for sharing your lives and your precious children with me.
May you be free to care for yourselves as fully as you care for others.

CONTENTS

Part Three

UNDERSTANDING THE COMPLEXITIES OF FEMALE CHEMISTRY

Yes! Mom's Health Matters!

It was a typical afternoon in my office, right after lunch. As I picked up the manila-colored chart of my next patient, I heard a voice coming from behind the exam room door. "Stay up there, Joshua. Dr. Carter will be here in just a minute." I tapped on the door and walked in to find three-year-old Joshua; his mother, Beth; five-year-old sister, Emily; and eighteen-month-old brother, Jacob.

"Hello, everyone! Well hello, Joshua! Look at you up there like a big boy!"

Joshua sat on the crinkled paper atop the exam table, wearing only his socks and underwear and flashing a beaming grin.

"Hi, Dahk-tor Cah-ter! I here for a checkup," Joshua announced, "but I haff a cold in my nose."

Joshua was in for his yearly physical, but the whole group looked a bit under the weather—especially his mother. I had met Beth six years earlier during a prenatal interview when she was pregnant with Emily and had cared for each of her kids from birth on.

On this day, Beth looked particularly tired. "Since it's spring break, I have the whole crew with me today. And we *all* have colds," said Beth with a sigh.

As I thoroughly checked Joshua, we talked about his growth and development, diet, and preschool. Emily sat cross-legged on the floor, absorbed in a book, while Jacob gave up trying to open the cabinet doors and instead pulled everything out of Beth's wallet and scattered it like confetti.

After we finished talking about Joshua's health, I asked Beth, "Now, how are *you* doing?"

"Well, okay," she said.

Not really convinced, I prodded her to continue.

"I love being a mom, and I don't want to complain, but since Joshua has been in preschool and Emily in kindergarten, I have been sick more times than they have! And since this last pregnancy, I can't seem to get my energy back. I'm so tired all the time. Maybe I need some vitamins. Plus, I still can't fit back into my old clothes—even though I'm running around all the time. It's so frustrating."

Beth looked more discouraged than I had ever seen her. "Have you made it to your doctor recently?" I asked.

"No, there never seems to be time, and our health insurance just changed so I don't even know who to go to. I'll be all right."

"How's your marriage?" I asked. "Are you and Bill getting out on any dates—just the two of you?"

Beth shook her head. "No, not really. We don't have any family in town and a sitter for three kids is pretty expensive—especially since I haven't gone back to work since Jacob was born. We use all of our time trying to keep up with the kids."

As a pediatrician in practice for over ten years, I talked with moms all day long. My heart goes out to Beth—and all mothers, because nearly every day I spent in my office, I heard similar concerns from moms. Moms with questions about personal health issues such as the following:

- How do I get more energy?
- What are healthy weight-loss programs that work?
- What nutritional supplements should I be taking?

- When is it normal "baby blues" and when is it a more serious form of depression?
- Who is the right doctor for me? For my children?

Many moms are like Beth. They give their very best to meet the needs of their family and end up with too little time or energy to take good care of their own needs. As a doctor I have learned that the well-being of a mother is not separate from the well-being of a child; a mother's needs and her child's needs intimately affect each other. One of the most important things a mother can do for her child is to take excellent care of herself—this is care for her family as well!

If Beth's dilemma sounds familiar, this book was written for you. Can you relate to giving as much as you can to be the best mom you can be? Is there too little time and energy left to meet *your* needs? If a close friend of yours confided in you that she felt the way Beth does, wouldn't you advise her to take better care of herself? Well, you deserve the same caring advice.

So what is keeping you from caring for your *own* health in the way you would advise a close friend? I understand that it is not easy to take care of everyone else's needs plus your own. For twelve years I, like you, have been trying to be the best mother I can be to a wonderful and very active son while trying to balance home, work, and personal health demands. It has been tough—at times impossible—to find the right balance. And the part of life that has suffered the greatest neglect is my own health. Ironically, when this has happened, every other area of life that I work so hard to protect has suffered. I want to help you avoid this trap. I want to help you make wiser decisions about your health needs. *Caring for yourself is a family priority!*

Does It *Really* Matter?

But it's not just an issue of selfishness, is it? With so much begging for your immediate attention, it's just easier to put your own health on a back burner if you don't have a known health problem. In fact, many moms have told me, "I'm young and healthy. There isn't really a need for me to worry about my health since I don't have any health problems." So—are they right? Does it really matter?

Health magazine, in its 2001 "Women in Motion" study, asked more than 3,000 women when they started to put their health first. The average age given was thirty-five, and the number-one reason was "When I developed a health problem."[1] For some women the wake-up call was high blood pressure or high blood cholesterol. Others realized their long-term habit of *not* exercising finally had caught up with them, and they no longer had the energy or stamina they needed for their daily life. Others, like Sandi Lloyd, were suddenly faced with a major disease, such as heart disease or multiple sclerosis, and were forced to reevaluate the stress, work habits, and the lifestyle they live. Says Sandi,

> I was diagnosed with multiple sclerosis in 1992: The diagnosis devastated me. I was working full time and caring for a young child while my husband was on the road. I wasn't eating right or exercising regularly.... One day I woke up in excruciating pain and could barely move; the symptoms were related to MS. That was the defining moment for me. I had to make some changes in my life, and I had to start making my health a priority.[2]

Why do we feel we need to wait until we already have a problem? Even though we are "super moms," we are not invincible! Not taking caring of your own health has consequences. For instance, it has been proven that high stress for a long period of time greatly increases your risk of getting a serious illness in the not-so-distant future. Do you want to take that risk?

Please take a moment and ask yourself this question: *What will happen to my family if I become seriously ill?* (Perhaps the thought crossed your mind that being sick might actually be a bit of a relief from all that you have to do and be.) The reality of being an ill parent is not something you would welcome. There are mothers who manage this challenge with amazing success, but it is very difficult. On a "good day" when you are ill, you likely will have less energy and ability to function than you used to have on a "bad day." And the day-to-day demands of family life continue even when you cannot keep up with them.

I know all too well the difficulties of being an ill mother. While driving to work on a Friday morning in September 1999, my normal life came to a screeching halt when I became suddenly and seriously ill with Ménière's disease. One minute I was driving and feeling perfectly well; the next minute I couldn't see because the world in front of me was spinning frantically like a pinwheel in a fierce wind. A few days later, after many tests and consultation with many good doctors, I was diagnosed with Ménière's disease, a disease of the inner ear, the part of the ear that controls our balance. Every day since that fateful morning I have had constant mild dizziness, severe spells of dizziness called vertigo, and extreme fatigue. I also suffered some hearing loss. Because of my symptoms, I can no longer drive, can no longer work in my medical practice, and am often housebound (which makes picking up my son from school impossible; I thank God for my friends who gladly bring him home). No matter how I feel, my family still needs me every day. My son needs me to be as involved as possible in his life. Every day he still needs help with homework, and there are stories to be heard, school activities to attend. I love being a mom and taking care of my son, but as wonderful as these tasks are, they are so much more difficult to accomplish since I became ill. So you see, I have personal as well as professional reasons for wanting to help you be as healthy as you can.

My illness is one that I probably could not have prevented. And there are many other illnesses and medical conditions that, even if you take care of yourself, are impossible to prevent. But what about those health problems we *can* prevent or at least delay? Wouldn't it be worth it to make even a few small changes in your lifestyle? You could be healthier, live longer, and feel better. If you said yes—or even maybe—then this is the book for you!

Have you ever dreamed of getting away to a luxurious health spa where you could leave it all behind for a while? Consider this book a retreat to a caring health spa—a place where my wish is to pamper you and bring you to the best state of health possible. A place where you can just be yourself. A place where you will have the time and permission to get your life into a new and healthier state of balance. A place where you are treated as the unique, amazing woman that you are, because you deserve it!

While relaxing at the "MOPS Health Spa," we will look at a wide range of different health issues for moms. All of these issues were topics found to be important to the moms surveyed in the MOPS Moms Health Survey. I have brought into the "spa" several consulting experts from different fields of women's health, and they will share their expertise with you. You will also receive practical tips on how to put this knowledge to work right away to improve your health. Together we'll tackle some of the most common personal health questions submitted by moms just like you.

Your health is comprised of four interconnected components: physical, mental, emotional, and spiritual. Since this is a "full-service spa," we will touch on all four components in the chapters ahead. Please give yourself the gift of this "trip to the health spa," even if it's only a few pages at a time. This book was written for you. It is less expensive than a day at a usual spa, but could be much more valuable to you if you take advantage of all its offerings. So it's up to you. Why not slip into your comfy spa slippers and robe and let the pampering begin? Why? Because you and your health matter!

The MOPS Moms Health Survey: What You Wanted to Know about Your Health

What do you want to know about your health? That's what *I* wanted to know. This book is especially for you—the woman you are, the mother you are, the *everything* you are! The MOPS Moms Health Survey was created and placed on the MOPS website so you could tell us what you want to know. Your answers and questions were gathered over a two-month time period. Thank you to all who participated! Your responses helped shape the direction and content of this book, which was designed to meet your specific needs and answer many of your questions.

The Survey

The survey had three sections:

1. The first asked moms to write in their "biggest health issue right now."
2. The second asked moms to rank fourteen different health issues in order of importance to them personally.

3. The third gave moms the chance to ask the doctor up to three questions about their health.

The fourteen health issues moms were asked to rank were:

Need for More Energy
Stress Reduction
Proper Nutrition
Weight-Loss Plans
Vitamins
PMS
Other Nutritional Supplements
Menopause
Feeling Overwhelmed
Feeling Depressed
Heart Attacks
Strokes
Diabetes
Staying Healthy When Your Kids Are Sick

The responses revealed some interesting information: Overwhelmingly, the biggest issue for moms surveyed was *the need for more energy*.

The five most important issues given (in order of most responses per issue):

1. Need for More Energy
2. Weight-Loss Plans
3. Feeling Overwhelmed
4. Stress Reduction
5. Proper Nutrition

The top ten issues for moms surveyed, based on the questions they asked, were:

1. Energy
2. Weight Related
3. Safe Birth Control
4. Libido/Sex Drive
5. Stress
6. Menopause
7. Vitamins and Herbs
8. Skin Health
9. Exercise
10. Cholesterol

Do any of these match the concerns on your list?

We will get to every one of these issues in the chapters that follow. I'll also share some interesting tidbits that came up when I analyzed the survey results. And, as promised, there are answers to the questions most frequently asked by those surveyed.

This book is all about moms just like you finding out what they *want to know* about taking care of their own health. As a doctor, I've added information on a few other health topics, which is information you *need to know* to ensure your good health. Together we'll discover how to achieve good health to help us feel better and be even better moms. So let's get started with the issue most requested by our surveyed moms—*the need for more energy!*

Part One

Solve Your Personal Energy Crisis

1

Your Personal Energy Crisis

Battling fatigue and needing more energy is the number-one issue for the moms we surveyed: 34 percent ranked it in first place, and 64 percent listed this issue as one of their top three concerns! Are you experiencing any "rolling blackouts," times when your energy runs out before the day does? If you are, you're not alone. Researchers at Cornell University found that parents with two children spend an average of 57,661 hours—almost eight hours a day—raising them to age eighteen, with more hours per day spent when the children are younger than age six.[1] You give, give, give, *give* every day as a parent. No wonder you need more energy! Here at the "MOPS Spa," we'll help you find solutions to relieve your energy crisis. But to find the right solutions, let's first look at *why* you are so tired.

The Hardest Job in the World

Parenting may be the hardest job in the world. There are no other jobs that require you to stay committed for the rest of your life and, for nearly two decades, require you to be on the job or on call 24 hours a day, 365 days a year! Here's the job description for being a parent:

- Meet the physical needs of your children (feeding, clothing, cleaning), which at the beginning is a 24-hour-a-day job.
- Care for your children's emotional needs (to be loved, encouraged, held, and nurtured), which constantly change as the children grow and mature.
- Train your children in spiritual and moral matters.
- Teach your children about the world and ensure that they are being properly educated, through school studies and in the home.
- Watch closely the behavior of your children and apply discipline as needed.
- Play with your children.
- Be there for your children whenever they need you, even sacrificing your sleep whenever necessary to care for your children's needs.

In her book *A Mother's Heart,* Jean Fleming offers a great way to look at the role of a mother:

> I enjoy the breadth of the challenge. The task of mothering can be as broad as I make it. Consider the endless variety of jobs a mother may do: teacher, nurse, dietitian, psychologist, chauffeur, trainer, disciplinarian, seamstress, baseball coach, interior decorator.[2]

Of course, it is an understatement to say that the benefits of parenting are better than any other job. Who could ever have adequately explained to you how deeply you would love this little child? It is beyond any choice of words! This love is the fuel that enables us to do all we must do for our children, and it is higher in octane than any other love we've ever experienced! This love of mother for a child makes us

> *"Why am I so tired all the time? How can I get more energy?"*

keep going even when we are exhausted. This love is so strong we would lay down our own lives for our children.

Well, "laying down our own lives" is what most of us find we have to do—to some degree—to make motherhood work. Temporarily you may have to let go of your expectations about having a spotless house, or having a to-do list that gets fully checked off by the end of each day, or being able to stay up until the wee hours and then sleep in the next day to recover.

When you start to feel discouraged about the difficulties of mothering, and just plain exhausted from all that you do, please remember that what you are doing as a mother *is very important!* As Jean Fleming writes,

> The aspect of mothering that excites me the most is knowing I am making a permanent difference in my children's lives. I am a woman of influence. I impart values, stimulate creativity, develop compassion, modify weaknesses, and nurture strengths. I can open life up to another individual. And I can open an individual up to life.[3]

Because your job is so important, we need practical ways to maximize your energy level. There are two basic keys to maintaining enough energy to make motherhood work:

1. Find out what is depleting your personal energy supply.
2. Make smart choices to manage and increase your energy supply.

What Causes Energy Depletion?

Let's cover the most common reasons for energy depletion so you can pick out what drains your personal energy supply.

1. *Exhaustion with no time to recuperate.* I think we all fit under this one. Actually, this statement would fit nicely in Webster's definition of "mother."
2. *Worry and stress.* Perhaps the biggest worries parents have concern their children. And it makes sense! God has given

you the most precious earthly gift one could ever imagine, along with all the responsibility to take care of that gift and the desire to cherish it. The flip side is that we usually feel a great burden to do it right and a fear that we will do it wrong.

3. *Emotional investment in our children.* Who knows better how to push your buttons? The good news is that your children push your "love" buttons the way no one else ever has. The not-so-good news is they can push your anger, fear, and hurt buttons with the same finesse. This emotional roller coaster is exhausting.
4. *Need for more spiritual renewal time.* When you are the parent of a young child, interruptions always seem to happen right in the middle of a quiet time or church service.
5. *Improper nutrition.* You're very concerned about how your children eat, but how about your own diet? You may not be refueling your body with the food and nutrients you need.
6. *Excess weight and radical diet plans.* Many moms feel sluggish because of excess weight and then try dieting aids and plans that may further deplete their energy supply.
7. *Lack of exercise.* There are so many ways that exercise can boost your energy level, but you won't enjoy the results if you don't work out.
8. *Sleep deprivation.* Sleep experts recommend at least seven hours of sleep each night to maintain good health. But according to a recent study, employed mothers reported they were getting less than six hours of sleep per night, and stay-at-home mothers averaged six hours of sleep per night.[4] Sleep deprivation is a *huge* issue for a majority of moms. Let's look at it now.

Will I Be Sleep Deprived Forever?

Nearly every mother I know has found that her expectations of what motherhood would be like did not quite match the reality. The always angelic child who sleeps in her bassinet on command is not what we get. One of the biggest myths of pre-motherhood is the assumption that we will be *well rested* when we are mothers. Even if friends and family warned that mothers are up in the middle of the night—every night—for the first several months of a child's life, most of us did not have a true understanding of how sleep deprivation colors our whole motherhood experience. Until we get there.

> *"I really need about seven hours of sleep a night, but I'm lucky to get six hours. It's not my baby's fault, because she sleeps between eleven and twelve hours a night. It's just that I stay up and try to get so much done while she is sleeping. That way when she's up I can give 100 percent of my attention to her—especially since I have her in daycare."*
>
> *—Joanne, mother of an eighteen-month-old child*

I thought my medical internship and residency were the hardest things in the world—until I became the mother of a newborn. Instead of being on call every third night and then coming home to sleep, as a new mom I found myself on call every night, breastfeeding at least twice in the middle of the night, with no chance to catch up on sleep! Sleep deprivation affects how well our brains function to how easily we become irritable to how susceptible we become to illness. Plus, it feels awful to be so tired. Being a mom is so much more difficult (and less enjoyable) when you are very tired, sick, or discouraged! And if you're a mom who had your children in your late thirties or even older, sleep deprivation likely will hit you harder than it does moms in their twenties.

Sleep deprivation is not solely a condition of moms of infants. Moms of kids of all stages and ages are notorious for staying up late trying to get "everything" done, only to find themselves overtired when morning comes and the duties start all over again.

What Is Your Level of Energy Depletion?

Mothers need two types of renewal to solve their personal energy crisis. They need to be *refreshed* and *replenished.* These are two very different kinds of help.

Refreshment includes the little moments when you can recharge your batteries. When you are working twenty-four hours a day—even when it is in this amazing job of parenting, working with those you love more than anyone else—you need breaks. So many of us forget to take these breathers, especially when we work in the home full-time. Please respect your need for these refreshing breaks and find little snatches of time to de-stress, change your focus, and have a quiet time, even if it's only five minutes at a time.

Replenishment is a more significant kind of renewal. If there were such a thing as an energy station for people to replenish, we'd be hooked up to energy IVs that would flow energy full blast into both arms! As mothers we often feel used up, and we are when we give and give and give but do not put back into ourselves what we pour out. Many moms have a faulty notion that they are like magic wishing wells. They think that no matter how much they dip in and pull out there is always, magically, an abundant supply. (This belief is probably due in part from watching certain Disney movies over and over again with our kids!) Although our God *is* magical and can do all things, he made each of us human, with physical, mental, and emotional limits. We need

> *"How do you take care of yourself and the baby at the same time?"*

refreshment and replenishment on a regular basis. Are you now in the need for refreshment, or do we need to hook you up to the replenishment pumps?

Smart Energy Management

Energy is a funny thing. It can either increase or decrease based on what we do physically, spiritually, emotionally, and intellectually. Likewise, our energy supply is also affected by all that is done to us, like the draining effect the unexpected flood from a broken pipe had on you, or the days when no matter what you do, your child pushes every limit, and you are beyond your point of exhaustion. With the unpredictability of all these forces, how can we hold onto the supply of energy we need? Certainly there is much you cannot change about the unpredictability of mothering, or life for that matter. But there are smart choices you *can* make that will help you weather the storms as they come and give you a buffer against the energy drain. You *can* increase your energy, and you *can* manage the energy you have.

> *"I could be more productive if I would just get to bed on time. I think I would still get everything done."*
>
> *—Patricia, mother of a six year old and three-year-old twins*

Often the best thing you can do when you are overwhelmed, exhausted, and cannot see the forest for the trees is to step back and look at the situation from a bird's-eye view. Ask yourself these three questions:

- What is really important in this situation?
- Is there something I can change that will make this better?
- What can I be grateful for in spite of this situation?

One of the best things you can do to reenergize and relieve stress is to choose to exercise gratitude. There is *always* something to be thankful for, and I promise that if you look for it, you will feel better.

Then consider the following two options:

1. *Change life habits.* Many moms, like Patricia, find that choosing to temporarily give up some old life habits is key to a happier time in the midst of motherhood. This is part of laying down your own life for your child. For those of you who are like Patricia, this may mean choosing to go to bed earlier even if it means the laundry isn't folded yet and the dinner dishes are still in the sink. What life habits could you change in order to be more rested?
2. *Find what energizes you.* Energy, like time, is a finite resource, so often you must decide what you really need to do and let the rest go. But energy is also an unusual resource in that doing something you really enjoy gives you more energy. What are those energizing things for you? Laughing at a joke or funny movie? Reading a humorous story? Exercising? Sharing a cup of tea with a friend? Having a quiet time of Bible study and prayer? Jot down all the ideas that come to mind.

It's Your Choice

You have a choice. You can take time out when you are spent, or choose not to and resent. If we do not stop to rest, relax, refresh, and replenish ourselves, then we will resent our children and regret our responses.

Keep in mind that there are valid reasons why you are so tired and lack energy. Let this confirmation bring you peace of mind. But I want you to have more than peace of mind; I wish you refreshment, replenishment, and a new perspective on your life as a mom. But where do we find these treasures? Through our relationship with God, the fellowship and support of family and friends, and sometimes even professional counseling, we can find replenishment. And through personal factors like diet and exercise and stress management we can find healthier, more functional ways to thrive as moms.

In the next five chapters we will take a detailed look at the common personal factors that either deplete or boost your energy supply: stress and anxiety, diet, use of nutritional supplements, weight control, and exercise. As we examine how each of these factors affects your life, you will get "personalized spa treatment." So take heart. Many specific and practical solutions are waiting for you in the pages ahead.

2

Stress and Anxiety Reduction for Moms on the Run

Stress Is Hard to Avoid

The day did not start out well. I was awakened by a painfully early call from an overly zealous solicitor, only to realize I had a migraine headache. It had been a rough night with my son, Robert, who kept waking up because of a viral illness. Unfortunately, the phone also woke Robert, who was tired and cranky.

"All I want is pancakes" was his answer as I prodded him to *eat something* for breakfast. He had eaten very little since becoming ill with the virus, so I grabbed the mix, eggs, milk, and oil. "Let's use that new pancake pan," I said with more enthusiasm than I felt. I should have known better than to try out a new contraption on a morning like this, but I did anyway because I wanted to be a fun mom. As I flipped the Perfect Pancake pan over with its inaugural pancake, batter poured out the sides and ran all over the electric burner and the stove top. I tried to mop it up quickly, but the batter was already frying on the burner, sending up a cloud of smoke. Then the smoke alarm went off, which is about the worst sound to hear when you have a migraine! Our dog started howling at the screeching smoke alarm . . . and the pancake burned to a blackened crisp. Just when I thought the moment couldn't get more stressful, my son ran in from the garage where he had gone to escape the piercing alarm. "MOMMMYYYY!" he yelled. "There's water all over the garage!" I looked at the front door and, for an instant, wondered if running away was an option. . . .

Have you ever felt so stressed and exhausted that you, the mother, just wanted to run away from home? You are not alone. Even the most devoted Christian moms get stressed out, pooped out, and at some moments want to get out. But like all the other on-the-run moms, you don't really want to run away permanently, you just need effective ways to escape the stress and anxiety that seem inescapable at times in motherhood.

So now is your time at the spa to take a break and let us help you understand

- Why you are stressed,
- What the consequences are of being stressed,
- How you can prevent some of your stress, and
- Practical solutions to help you cope with stress you can't prevent.

(And our solutions include more than just massages.)

It's Time to Unearth the "Whys"

Stress and anxiety are exhausting and the last thing you need on top of the hectic life of caring for a family. You know it is important to get your stress and anxiety under control as much as possible. But it doesn't work to just tell yourself, "I will no longer be stressed or anxious," does it? To truly manage stress and anxiety, we must first understand the causes. We need to dig to the roots of the stressful feelings and unearth them. Then we can figure out the best strategies to prevent unnecessary stress and to deal with the stress and anxiety we cannot prevent.

When Your Expectations Collide with Reality

Many moms give birth daily to the undesirable offspring named "Stress" and "Anxiety." This usually happens whenever their expectations collide with reality. This conflict produces stress and anxiety and leads to feelings of being overwhelmed. For many moms this mismatch of expectations and reality happens often, even daily! Take a moment and reflect on your premotherhood expectations about

- What you would be like as a mother,
- How your children would behave, and
- How difficult or easy mothering would be.

I suspect you see some major mismatches between how you thought motherhood would be and how it really is. These mismatches can give rise to some pretty ugly feelings we will call the "Six Ugly Stepsister Emotions of Mothering." We would all like to ignore them and pretend they don't exist, but they do exist and need to be addressed. And more moms deal with these same thoughts and feelings than you may imagine! So let's get them out in the open. Can you identify with these thoughts and feelings?

1. *Fear:* "Will my kids turn out all right? Am I doing this right?"
2. *Anger:* "Why is mothering so much harder than I expected?"
3. *Guilt:* "I have to leave them so much. Am I a good enough mom?"
4. *Worry:* "Are my children safe at home? At school? At daycare?"
5. *Resentment:* "I'm trying so hard. Why does my child make it so hard for me to be a good mom? Why won't my husband help out more?"
6. *Sadness:* "I wish I could enjoy my children and my life more."

Exposing the Myths of Motherhood

These emotions are normal human responses, so if you recognize them in yourself, don't start beating yourself up for experiencing them. It is understandable to react this way because deep down you know motherhood is the most important job you will have in your life. Your children are the most precious beings in the world to you, and you feel completely responsible for their safety, their growth, and for helping them become all that God intends them to be. So of course you want to do it right. All these emotions—and the stress and anxiety that come with them—come from the root emotions of fear and anger. Both fear and anger are present *because* we want to do this right, and because we believe that how we "mother" directly affects how this child will turn out. But we can control only some of the things about ourselves, our children, and what happens in the rest of the world. Many of us find that we fall short of being the ideal mothers we thought we would be.

So how can we change this vicious cycle? You are already taking the first step by identifying what your motherhood expectations really are. An excellent tool to guide you and help you evaluate your expectations is the MOPS book *Real Moms: Exploding the Myths of Motherhood* by Elisa Morgan and Carol Kuykendall. Here is an excerpt from this candid and practical book:

> Welcome to the reality of motherhood—a bumpy, wonderful, self-revealing, growing place where a woman faces the constant tension between expectations and reality. Between good-mom myths and real-mom truths.[1]
>
> Are you tired of constantly trying—and failing—to be a perfect mom? Stop beating yourself up and let the truth about motherhood set you free! *Real Moms* debunks the "good mom" fallacies that have weighed you down by giving you some liberating "real mom" truths. This book punctures such mother myths as:
>
> - Good moms look good all the time.
> - Good moms keep everybody happy.

- Good moms instinctively know what their children need.
- Good moms take responsibility for how their children turn out.
- Good moms don't admit their feelings of guilt or anger or fear—because to admit those feelings might make them like they are not good moms.[2]

Good-mom myths pressure us to be something we can't be and don't need to be, something beyond what we were intended to be. The truth sets us free to be honest and growing and vulnerable.

Good-mom myths fill us with impossible "I shoulds." Truth allows us to focus on the "I ams."

Good-mom myths give us idealistic formulas and unrealistic expectations from a "once upon a time" and happily ever after" perfect world of make-believe. But we don't live there. We are imperfect people living in the midst of imperfect relationships, trying to do our best, while juggling busy schedules on PMS and bad hair days. In the midst of this reality, we can discover personal growth and contentment as we seek to know the truth and to act like we believe the truth. That takes hard work and sometimes feels risky, but the results are worth the effort.

It's time to explode the myths of motherhood with the truth that will set you free to be the best mom you can be.[3]

- Free to quit trying to be so good all the time.
- Free to acknowledge that there are no perfect families in this world, and no perfect children and no perfect mothers.
- Free to admit where we fall short of our own expectations or someone else's.
- Free to not feel guilty about not being good enough or home enough or fun enough or patient enough.
- Free to become all God created us to be.[4]

What Myths Are You Living Under?

Now it's time to check your expectations against the motherhood "myths list" and "truths list." How many of your personal expectations show up on the first list? It's time to change your expectations to meet the needs of your new reality. As you think through your personal expectations, it helps to know *how* they came to be. These expectations come from a few common sources:

- How we were raised
- What we see other mothers say and do
- Messages from the experts through books, TV and radio, and our own doctors
- Our basic personality or temperament

Your Personality Factor

Your basic personality or temperament impact your mothering and personal expectations more than you may realize. It affects the expectations we place on ourselves and how we react to those put upon us by others. It also can affect whether we feel stressed or anxious in the first place. Risa, a longtime mom of a patient of mine, shook her head in exasperation while in my office one day, lamenting, "I just can't keep from worrying about Timmy, no matter how hard I try! I get so frustrated at home. I guess it's just my nature." Risa is the mother of a busy little boy as well as a corporate executive at a prestigious company. She makes things run smoothly in the company and checks off all the "to-dos" on her list before going home each workday. But at home, life cannot be controlled in the same fashion. On this day Risa was especially frustrated because she had just visited her sister, a stay-at-home mother of four active children who seems to glide above the stress of motherhood and never appears to worry. Why? Because her sister's *nature* is to be laid back and not be bothered by the chaos around her.

You've likely heard about the longtime debate of *nature* versus *nurture,* which poses the question: How much of our behavior is affected by our genetics and how much is affected by the environment we live in? Of course, both influence how we act and who we are, but when it comes to personality, much of the die is cast before we greet the bright lights of this world with our first wail.

Some moms can let tasks go undone more naturally than others. You probably have seen these moms. Take for example the mom who has five children all busy at play and running around the house and yard, and yet she is able to sit, smiling, cool as a cucumber, enjoying and even joining in the chaos around her. For those of us who are *not* naturally that way, please understand that it is likely you were born with a different temperament or personality than these cool-as-a-cucumber moms.

There are four basic temperaments or personalities, and nearly all of us are predominantly a combination of two: a main temperament and a minor temperament. See if you recognize yourself in these brief descriptions:

1. *Perfect Melancholy.* Quieter, deeper, more thoughtful. You strive for perfection in your life and are often disappointed and tend toward depression because perfection in life is rarely if ever attained. Your catchphrase: "If it is worth doing it is worth doing right."
2. *Powerful Choleric.* Can be bossy and short-tempered. But on the positive side, you are goal oriented, highly organized, a high achiever, and very outgoing. Your catchphrase: "Just do it!"
3. *Popular Sanguine.* High energy, happy, fun-loving, very social, and outgoing. You can be disorganized and forgetful of details and obligations. You are not happy when you are not having fun. Your catchphrase: "Are we having fun yet?"
4. *Peaceful Phlegmatic.* Peaceful, relaxed, easygoing, and steady. This is the most contented and balanced of the four temperament types. You may appear to be lazy and lack

drive or motivation. Your catchphrase: "Why stand when you can sit, and why sit when you can lie down?"[5]

According to Marita Littauer, a personality expert, teacher, and author of multiple books on personality types,

> There are definitely some personality types that deal with stress better than others. There are some that internalize it more and there are some that verbalize it more. Those that internalize their stresses are the ones who have a harder time with the stress (Melancholy and Choleric), versus those who are very vocal about what is going on (Sanguine and Phlegmatic).[6]

Does this mean we are stuck with the constraints of our personality types? Are some of us doomed to a life of worry and stress? No! Once we know the limitations of our temperaments, we can learn ways to overcome these natural tendencies.

For a clearer picture of which temperaments fit your true nature, as well as the strengths and weaknesses that are yours, I highly recommend the following sources:

The Personality Profile. This is a simple, low cost ($1 each) test you can easily take and score at home, available from CLASServices at 1-800-433-6633, www.thepersonalities.com, or P.O. Box 66810, Albuquerque, NM 89193-6810.

Getting Along with Almost Anybody: The Complete Personality Book by Florence and Marita Littauer. This book contains the Personality Profile, plus advice on how to use your understanding about temperaments to help you get along better with your children, spouse, coworkers, etc. (also available from CLASServices or in bookstores).

Children Have Temperaments Too!

Another big source of stress is the clashing of your temperament with your *child's* natural temperament. Plus, if you have more than one child, each one has his or her own temperament, so this can translate into some wild family dynamics. And just when you think you have discipline figured out for one child, you may find that the same technique does not work with the temperaments of the other children. Whew! I recommend Florence Littauer's book *Personality Plus for Parents* for those of you on this wild ride.

Hormone Havoc

Another major cause of exhausting stress and anxiety is the fluctuation of female hormones, which happens during PMS, pregnancy, and perimenopause (the five to ten years leading to menopause). Yes, there are *real reasons* you feel so many unpleasant symptoms during these times. In chapter 16 we will look in more detail at what you can do to decrease these symptoms and the stress, anxiety, and fatigue that come with them.

The Stresses of Stay-at-Home-to-Work Moms vs. Go-to-Work Moms

Whether you are a mom who does her work at home full-time with the kids or a mom who goes to work outside of the home, you have some of the same stresses in common. But each group has its own unique set of stresses. Neither one has it "easy."

Stay-at-home-to-work moms have less adult contact, which they may especially miss if they had a career prior to choosing to stay at home. Those who worked outside the home before may also feel like they lack identity that comes with a job title, especially if they hear the occasional "What *else* do you do?" comment. Since there is only one income, there is often less in financial resources. There are no scheduled coffee breaks or lunch hours since most at-home moms do not have a coworker nearby to relieve them during the day. Instead the at-home mom experiences the stress that comes with caring for children full-time, *all* the time! And even if you relish every minute of being there to raise your children, *you need breaks* (which your husband may or may not fully understand when he comes home from work at night).

Go-to-work moms are *not* part-time moms. All mothers—whether at home or at work during the day—are concerned and committed to their children *all* the time. And that is why it is very stressful for the go-to-work mom to juggle her priorities. As long as everything is going as planned, it is usually okay; but when her child gets sick, she must decide whether to miss work or trust someone else with her child's care. There is always pressure from work for the mom to be there and devote herself fully to the job, no matter what is going on at home. When home, she often tries to make up for the time spent away from her children. In addition to her work tasks, she still has all her household responsibilities unless she can hire someone to do some of these.

No mom has it easy; all have reasons to be stressed. That is a given. So where do we go from here? It is time to take a good look at why we need to decrease the stress in our lives and how we can best do just that.

Why Is Stress Such a Big Deal?

Stress isn't just draining and uncomfortable. Medical problems have been connected with stress. There are so many that we could fill whole pages of this book with them. Everything from headaches, back and neck spasms, and increased susceptibility to viral infections, as well as coronary artery disease and heart attacks, strokes, autoimmune diseases, plus Crohn's Disease and certain forms of arthritis all can be brought on or made worse by emotional stress. Let's face it, our bodies are trying to tell us that stress is not good for us.

Research shows us that chronic emotional stress is what we should be most concerned about. The most harmful combination of body chemicals, which include the hormones adrenaline (or epinephrine) and cortisol, is released with emotional stress, and the effect is made worse if the release happens over and over on a chronic basis.[7] What happens is your brain sends the emotional distress signal to your adrenal glands, telling them to pump out the stress hormones, which help you in the short term. But on a chronic basis, these chemicals overtax the brain, heart, lungs, and muscles. At the same time, they shut down less essential functions by shunting blood away from those areas. This spells trouble over the long haul. In addition, adrenaline causes chaos in the immune system, and cortisol tells the body to increase the sugar supply in the bloodstream for quick energy. This also turns on the cortisol fat-storing mechanism, which tells the fat cells in your abdomen to redeposit fat. That is why you gain that spare tire of fat around your midsection when you've been under a constant stream of stress. Even very lean women who are under chronic stress are often found to have this abdominal accumulation of fat.[8]

This type of fat accumulation spells danger for both women and men. Studies show that a buildup of internal abdominal fat is associated with a higher risk of heart attack, stroke, diabetes, and high blood pressure. It is also a key to recognizing those women with a dangerous condition known as *metabolic syndrome.* Women with metabolic syndrome have high blood pressure, high insulin levels, high blood lipid levels, and insulin resistance, which leads to high blood sugar levels.[9] How do you tell if you are at risk? One way is to measure your waist and your hips; if your waist measurement is 35 inches or greater (and you are not currently pregnant or did not recently have a baby), then you are at risk for metabolic syndrome. Or, if you divide the number of your waist measurement by your hips' measurement, you are at an increased risk if the result is 0.85 or greater (the waist-hip ratio). If you have reason for concern, consult your doctor right away.

Do you want to stop this ugly cycle of emotional stress? To do so you need to reach a state of relaxation that allows all these revved-up organs to take a load off, the hormone levels to decrease, and your body to return to normal operation. Now that you know what stress is doing to your body, let's look at the many effective ways we have to prevent and relieve our emotional stress and anxiety.

What to Do with Stress and Anxiety

What can we do to protect our bodies from stress? For starters, it is best to not compound the situation by choosing unhealthy ways to cope. As we will see in chapter 12, coping mechanisms like smoking, excessive eating, excessive shopping, alcohol and drug abuse, and extramarital affairs cause more problems than they solve. Exploding with rage at another person may seem slightly helpful at the time because you were able to vent your anger, but studies show that this kind of intense outward display of anger can lead to more stress and usually hurts relationships with others. Such explosions only give us more to feel guilty about and apologize for. Let's instead choose some healthier coping mechanisms.

Quick Rescue Techniques

When you feel like you are a pressure cooker that is just about to explode, you need help immediately! Why? Your body and mind are in a state that is biochemically destructive, and it will continue spiraling in that direction unless you intervene.

Just remember these three little words: *clear—quiet—breather.* First, you need to *clear* the area around you. If possible, move from the area where you are feeling stressed to an area with less stimulation, less clutter, and fewer demands. If you cannot physically move, then mentally transport yourself to another place that is peaceful and calming for you. You can do it even when you have a screaming two-year-old with you. It helps if you already have a mental picture of that calm place before you need to "go" there. Take a moment and think right now what would be the perfect spot for you.

Second, seek *quiet* if at all possible. Just stopping the stimulation on your eardrums and mind will help decrease your body's stress response. Quieting your mind is an important aspect of this part of your rescue. You cannot effectively solve anything when you're about to explode, so try to quiet all the chatter in your mind and concentrate only on your breathing.

This leads us to the third part of the rescue. Take a *breather* by doing a relaxation breathing exercise. You can do this simple breathing exercise anytime, anywhere, and it will have an immediate effect on your body. I call it the "4-by-4-by-4 Breather" exercise.

Step 1. Close your eyes (if possible). While mentally counting to four, take a slow, deep breath in through your nose so that your lower abdomen pushes outward. You may want to put your hand on your lower belly to be sure it moves outward.

Step 2. Hold this breath for another count of four; concentrate *only* on holding this breath.

Step 3. Gently release this breath so that it slowly flows out of your body through your mouth, again while counting to four.

Step 4. Repeat this exercise until you have done it at least four times in a row.

What is amazing about this breathing exercise is that it triggers relaxation in the processes of your body—slows your heart rate, relaxes your muscles, can even decrease your blood pressure, and quiets your mind. Great gains from such a simple tool!

The Tense-Release Sequence Exercise

Ready for the ultimate relaxing exercise? (You may wish to make an audiotape with this series of commands, so you can follow along and maximize your relaxation.)

- Sit on a chair or wherever you can sit upright with both feet flat on the ground. Close your eyes if you wish.
- Focus on what is happening with your muscles, but if stray thoughts come to your mind, do not fight them. Simply acknowledge them and let them drift back out.
- Do each of the following exercises twice and in order; tense each muscle for five seconds, then relax for about thirty seconds.

Exercise sequence:

1. Right hand and forearm (make a fist, then release)
2. Right upper arm (bend the arm and "show off your muscles," then release)
3. Left hand and forearm (make a fist, then release)
4. Left upper arm (bend the arm and "show off your muscles," then release)
5. Forehead (raise your eyebrows, then relax your face)
6. Eyes and cheeks (squeeze the eyes, then relax)
7. Mouth and jaw (clench your teeth and pull the corners of the mouth back, then relax)
8. Shoulder and neck (lock the fingers of both hands behind your neck and push your head back against this resistance, then relax and pull up your shoulders, letting them relax)
9. Chest and back (breathe in and hold a breath while you press your shoulders back, then relax your shoulders and breathe normally)
10. Belly (pull in abdomen muscles, then release)
11. Right-hand thigh ("shovel" right foot into floor but keep it in place, then release)
12. Right-hand calf (lift up just the heel, then release)
13. Right foot (curl the toes, then release)
14. Left-hand thigh ("shovel" left foot into floor but keep it in place, then release)
15. Left-hand calf (lift up just the heel, then release)
16. Left foot (curl the toes, then release)

After you finish all the exercises, breathe in deeply, then exhale while playfully wiggling your fingers and toes. Then take another deep breath. Exhale and stretch your whole body. Finally, breathe in deeply and open your eyes. Great job![10]

Head for the shower. One of the best places to escape to during a stress rescue is the shower. There is only "white" noise, you're in a fairly clear area, and the warm water will help your body to relax. If you close your eyes and do the 4-by-4-by-4 Breather exercise, you will quickly begin to feel better.

These quick interventions not only are useful for rescuing you when you are severely stressed, but if done on a regular basis (daily or several times a week), they will help to decrease the overall level of stress in your life.

Find Relief from Stress and Anxiety

Day-In-and-Day-Out De-Stressing

Make peace with your priorities. Earlier, when I suggested going to bed and, if need be, leaving the laundry unfolded and the dishes in the sink, perhaps you started feeling even *more* stressed and anxious. For many of you it is not your nature to leave work undone, but motherhood is a time when you need to weigh your priorities and see where the scale tips heavy. Which is more important: to have more energy available to be the mom you desire to be or to get all the housework finished? In theory, the answer is easy. We all want the energy to be better moms. But this is real life and we feel overwhelmed. Sometimes we just have to let some tasks go undone. Your peace of mind and your health are worth more than an empty laundry basket or a spotless kitchen. One of the biggest steps you can take toward having more energy and less stress is to make peace with your new priorities. When you find yourself getting anxious about all that is left to do, remember that the situation is temporary. Tell yourself, "This is only for a season, and there is a good reason." Once you've accepted your new priorities, and the pressure is off, you may find it easier to seek creative solutions to get the "left behind" tasks done, such as persuading your husband to pick up an additional specific duty. I will offer many other creative solutions later in this chapter.

Learn and respect your limits. No matter how much you do, whether you're a stay-at-home-to-work mom or a go-to-work mom, there will always be more that you could or "should" do. But each of us has limits—limits that need to be respected. Since you now know your new priorities, it is time you set your limits and stand firm. There will always be better meals to be made, optional letters to write, closets to be cleaned, worthy church and school activities, and extra projects at work. But there will not always be the chance to read your preschooler a story, the chance to nurture your child's budding faith in God, or the chance to sit and give your full attention when you answer questions like, "Why can't dogs fly?"

Doing it all is not what is important. Doing what is important while respecting your limits is what matters.

Take a break—have a timeout. When you become overly stressed and feel you need a timeout, take it! It's better for your child to hear you say, "Mommy needs a timeout," and see you walk away for a short time than end up in the path of your wrath. After your break, you will return more calm and able to handle that child.

When my son was a small infant, he had terrible colic for over four months. It was impossible to soothe him no matter what I did. I thought I would go out of my mind! How does a mother feel okay—or even neutral—when there is no way she can help her baby stop crying? At times the stress and anxiety bottled up inside me were so excessive that I had to do something immediately to relieve the pressure. At those times I would lay my screaming son down in his bassinet or hand him to my husband, then go out into our garage and climb into my fairly soundproof car. I would shut the car door and scream and yell at the top of my lungs! I also found that a physical release, such as hitting a big pillow, helped tremendously.

Brief distractions bring refreshment. Walk outside for a brief moment and notice the sky, really look at a beautiful picture, or listen to a song that inspires you. It is remarkable how these little things can help refresh your mind and spirit. What are your favorite distractions?

Don't worry, trust Jesus. Moms, it is completely understandable if you feel compelled to worry about your children and whether you are doing the right things as their mother. After all, you are their mother! But many of us worry too much, and that can damage our emotional, spiritual, and physical health. The chemicals released during an emotional stress response can cause serious physical damage. But it turns out that how we think we are handling a stressful situation affects how dangerous our emotional stress response is. If we are coping well, then the response will likely be less damaging.[11] So hold on to God's promises and perspective about your life and your children. Those promises will help you to hope and cope.

The best help and advice about worry comes from Jesus. First in Matthew 6:25–27:

> Therefore I tell you, do not worry about your life, what you will eat or drink; or about your body, what you will wear. Is not life more important than food, and the body more important than clothes? Look at the birds of the air; they do not sow or reap or store away in barns, and yet your heavenly Father feeds them. Are you not much more valuable than they? Who of you by worrying can add a single hour to his life?

Then in Matthew 6:34:

> Therefore do not worry about tomorrow, for tomorrow will worry about itself. Each day has enough trouble of its own.

There may be reasons behind your worry that extend beyond your immediate situation. Once we become mothers, issues about our own childhood or how we were parented can emerge frequently and without warning. For example, if you felt rejected by a parent, you may react very strongly to your baby "rejecting" you when you are trying to comfort or feed him or her. These old issues can dramatically color how you feel about your child and how you feel you are doing as a mom. They can make you feel depressed, angry, anxious, and very stressed. If this happens to you or someone you know, it is time to consult a trained Christian counselor. Depression can also be related to hormonal shifts. A qualified health professional can help sort out the underlying reason and help you get past it.

Whatever the reason, it is very important that you not feel you are alone. When you feel alone, stressed, anxious, and depressed, remember this: God loves you and is always with you. Think of all you would do for your child if he or she were in need. Then remember that you too have a parent, a heavenly Father, who cares for you *even more!* Just look at Matthew 7:9–11:

> Which of you, if his son asks for bread, will give him a stone? Or if he asks for a fish, will give him a snake? If you, then, though you are evil, know how to give good gifts to your children, how much more will your Father in heaven give good gifts to those who ask him!

As a follower of Christ, you have the assurance that God is with you each and every day, and that he cares for you and your family. He has a plan for your life. "'For I know the plans I have for you,' declares the Lord, 'plans to prosper you and not to harm you, plans to give you hope and a future'" (Jeremiah 29:11).

When everything is going wrong despite all your best efforts, you also have the assurance that God will work it all out in the end. Paul reminds us, "We know that in all things God works for the good of those who love him, who have been called according to his purpose" (Romans 8:28).

Raising children requires much more than just our strength and wisdom. And, thankfully, we don't have to do it alone! God is our willing and constant partner in parenting. "Trust in the Lord with all your heart and lean not on your own understanding; in all your ways acknowledge him, and he will make your paths straight" (Proverbs 3:5–6).

God wants to hear your concerns, your questions, and your needs—nothing is too small to bring before him. He is faithful to meet your needs and bring you peace. "Do not be anxious about anything, but in everything, by prayer and petition, with thanksgiving, present your requests to God. And the peace of God, which transcends all understanding, will guard your hearts and your minds in Christ Jesus" (Philippians 4:6–7).

Trust your radar and trust God. As a doctor and fellow mom, I want to reassure you about a few things. First, you *do* have internal radar about your children. You should trust your instincts. Countless times in my years as a pediatrician I have had moms bring their children in just because they "knew" something was not right, and countless times I found that these moms were right.

Yet even with your internal radar, you won't always know what to do for your children, and that is okay. God has not left you alone in this lifelong task of raising your children. He is always available to listen to your fears, your frustrations, and your requests for help. He also works through those around you who can listen and help you gain perspective and support when you need them. So trust your instincts and count on God to know what to do.

Check out your thinking and keep your thinking in check. Often the questions randomly running through our minds are what make us feel so stressed and anxious.

- "Am I doing a good enough job?"
- "Will he turn out all right?"

The questions we keep asking ourselves can undermine our parenting confidence. When you recognize them, face them head-on. Answer each one using the wisdom and confidence from God's promises:

- "I am doing the best job I can, and God is helping me."
- "God has a plan for each of my children, so I do not need to worry about how they will turn out."

Give yourself a dose of the grace that God gives you. We all blow it. But even when we lose our temper or react badly to stress, there is forgiveness and grace waiting for us in the arms of our heavenly Father. Give yourself the same measure of grace—forgive yourself. When you have reacted to your children or others in a way that you wish you hadn't, apologize to them and move forward. Our children need to see how we make amends so they will know how to make amends when they blow it. I have apologized to my eleven-year-old son so many times that he now says, nonchalantly, "Yeah, Mom, I know when you get mad that you're sorry. It's okay." And we move on.

Feed your spirit. Ideally, you need a daily quiet time for reading your Bible and for prayer as well as weekly times of church fellowship and worship. But for many moms these big blocks of time are impossible to find. Quick little "spirit snacks" can help tremendously:

- Play a local Christian radio station while you dress or do dishes.
- Sing worship songs.

- Use a Bible or devotional book with brief but powerful devotions, such as the *Mom's Devotional Bible: NIV*[12] or *Meditations for Mothers: Moments with God Amidst a Busy Nest* by Elisa Morgan.[13] Both are available at bookstores or directly from the MOPS International website: www.mops.org.
- Norman Vincent Peale's little booklet *Thought Conditioners* is perfect for busy moms because it highlights forty powerful verses with a brief comment on each. Take two minutes to meditate on one or more verses and let their power ease your anxiety and stress.[14]
- Pray throughout your day. Even right in the middle of your daily activities and challenges, you can talk to God. This invites God into everything we do. And he invites you to turn *everything* over to him and to tell him how you really feel.
- Use the church nursery, if possible, so you can have a worship and fellowship hour at church every Sunday. Many churches also have "cry rooms" where mothers of infants can go with their child and still hear the sermon. Or play tag team with your husband so you both get a chance to attend a worship service.
- Join a mothers' prayer group, such as Moms In Touch International at www.momsintouch.org, where you come together with other moms specifically to pray for your children, their schools, your families, and others in need.

Turn down the volume. Be aware of the overall effect that noise has on you. Having children around is noisy. They run. They slam doors. They scream and cry. They ask questions. Mix all that with the background sounds of TV and videos and the doorbell and the dialogue playing in your mind. It's no wonder you feel as though you can't think straight.

Streamline your tasks. With all the little things we need to do in addition to all the important tasks of motherhood that need our attention, we can easily feel overwhelmed. Even if it's not your nature to be super-organized, you will benefit from streamlining your everyday tasks. Here are some examples:

(1) To-do lists: A simple, ongoing to-do list can help you keep all the things you must do from overwhelming you. The main purpose of the list is to clear the nagging details from your mind by placing them in one place where you can find them whenever you have time to do something about them. Many moms use a small notebook for their to-do lists. Designate a place for the notebook and keep it there. You might tape it down so it won't wander away!

> Rule 1: Do not expect to clear the whole list off every day, or even every week.
>
> Rule 2: Keep the list simple.
>
> Rule 3: When you think of something—anything—you need to do, jot it down. (I draw a small box before each item on my list so I can check it off when the job is done. It shows me I am making progress!)

(2) Finances: Collect your bills as they arrive and put them in one designated place (a file slot or the pocket of a large organizer envelope). Pay them all on one designated day each month (or on two days if you pay twice a month). The day the bill arrives, make the bill ready to pay. Put the bill in its envelope and write discretely on the inside of the envelope flap the amount you need to pay. That way, on the designated day, you can grab your bundle of bills, write the checks, slip them into the prepared envelopes, add stamps, and mail them. Some credit card companies will permanently adjust your monthly due date if you request it. That way you can schedule all your bills to be paid at the same time. Also use pay-by-phone services that may be offered by your bank or creditors, automatic bill payment, and online banking services.

(3) Mail: Try to handle each piece of incoming mail only once. Toss it, recycle it, or place it in its designated slot or file. Bills in one spot (see above). Urgent correspondence that requires a reply in another. Letters from friends in another slot. Some moms put notecards and stamps in this same location so they can easily reply when they get a free moment.

(4) Shopping: Don't settle for just getting in and out of the grocery or department store. With kids in tow, shopping can be very stressful. Ease the stress by shopping while they sleep or play with supervision by Dad. Get what you need by phone or online. Some of the best online shopping resources are:

- *Grocery delivery sites:* These companies usually serve major cities and deliver groceries for a fee or free if you order a minimum dollar amount. Examples: www.albertsons.com, www.vons.com (West Coast U.S.), www.peapod.com (East Coast U.S.), and www.netgrocer.com (nationwide—delivery by FedEx, but with higher shipping costs because it's not a local service). If you type "grocery delivery" in your internet search box, and press Enter or Go or Search, you will see a list of current grocery delivery sites. In this business, companies often come and go, and delivery areas change, so check for the current companies in business in your area.
- *Drugstore sites:* These companies may be able to fill your prescriptions. They also carry a large selection of the usual personal and health care items. Two of the best sites are www.drugstore.com and www.savon.com.
- *"Everything Else" sites:* You can find nearly everything you need by shopping online. Some of the best shopping sites with reputable security are www.shopping.yahoo.com, www.amazon.com, www.iqvc.com, and www.hsn.com.

(5) Meals: Streamline meal preparation by cooking in bulk. In *Once-a-Month Cooking,* by Mimi Wilson and Mary Beth Lagerborg, the authors show you, step-by-step, how to take a weekend day once every few weeks and cook several dishes that you then package and freeze for quick, healthy dinners in the weeks to come. You may wish to do this with a friend. Either cook different recipes separately or make the cooking a social time, then split the meals, giving you twice the variety in your freezer.

(6) Cleaning: Learn how to clean your house in an hour, and other valuable tips. The "Fly Lady" gives a healthy perspective on cleaning and

keeping your house and your sanity at the same time via her website, www.flylady.net, and free daily email service. She takes you step-by-step through how to set up doable cleaning routines, get rid of clutter, and put your home and life in order. She sends this information through email reminders—multiple ones per day—but you can get the same information by going to her website. The Fly Lady divides the whole week's worth of cleaning into daily doable duties and will send you an email to remind you what to do each day. Some of her best bits of advice are to set a fifteen minute timer to do a task ("You can do anything for fifteen minutes") and to empty your kitchen sink before you go to bed each night so you feel a sense of accomplishment.

Get organized. Especially for those of you who thrive on having everything organized, I strongly recommend the book *Organizing from the Inside Out* by Julie Morgenstern.[15] This is the best book I've ever seen on organizing your life, designed for busy moms who may have only a few minutes at a time to read. It is practical, ingenious, and easy to follow, with step-by-step details (like what storage containers to use). It even works for those who aren't crazy about organizing!

Get by with a little help from your friends. Research confirms that women react differently to stress than men do. A woman's hormone response to stress makes her more likely to want to "tend and befriend." In other words, when stressed, a woman nurtures her children and seeks out friendship relationships with other women. This is in contrast to a man's usual hormonal response to stress that makes him more prone to "fight or flight." Put differently, a man will do battle against the stressor or run away from the stress.[16]

Now you have scientific support that is both natural and therapeutic for you to cope with stress by talking and socializing with other women friends! MOPS groups provide that outlet, and I encourage you to reach out to other moms and friends. A quick phone call or a walk around the block together with the kids in strollers can be not only enjoyable but therapeutic.

Accept help from your friends. Accept a meal or an offer of child care for your little ones, especially when you are in those seasons of mothering that are most taxing—when you've recently had a baby, much of the family is ill, or you're just having a hard time. You can return the favor at a later time or give some other type of help in the future. A friend who helps when you're in need is a special friend indeed!

Seek out humor to diffuse a stressful situation and find time to play. "You just gotta laugh or you'll cry" is a wise perspective when it comes to managing stressful situations. On countless occasions when stress is building, I have found humor the "healing elixir." Try to find the humor hiding in your stressful situations.

What makes you laugh? Research raves about the healthy benefits of laughing and playing. Studies show that just watching a thirty- to sixty-minute comedic video a day decreases the levels of the stress hormones in the blood. In one study with heart-attack patients, those who watched the videos had *five times fewer repeat heart attacks* than those patients who did not get this daily laugh therapy.[17] So grab the joke books, watch your favorite funny shows and movies, or make faces and be silly and giggle with your kids! Dancing in the living room to a fun song is also therapeutic for the whole family. Maybe it isn't your nature to bop around the living room, but that's precisely why you should try it. It will probably make you laugh. *Remember, a giggle a day helps keep the doctor away.*

What to *you* is "play"? Riding the roller coasters at Disneyland? Playing Scrabble? A game of golf? Reading *Wuthering Heights*? A crossword or logic puzzle? Whatever "play" is for you, find play that you can do. Then do it!

Find something to do with your body. The following measures directly decrease the unhealthy levels of the stress hormones adrenaline and cortisol:

- Exercise: *Whatever activity you will do, just do it!*
- Massage: *If you can, enlist your mate to do the honors.* If you are able to go for a professional massage, do! Research confirms what we already knew—massage relaxes muscles and reduces dangerous levels of stress chemicals in the bloodstream.
- Relaxing hot bath or shower: *Calgon . . . take me away!*

Live in the moment. Notice the comical way your daughter's hair mats on her forehead when you remove her hat. Take time to observe the intricacy of the city your son just built all over the living room floor. Delight with them when they see something for the first time. These moments help restore your soul.

Make time for your creative self. When you become a mother, it is often easier to let your personal interests drop into the diaper pail because of the overwhelming demands on your time and energy. But it doesn't have to be all or nothing. As MOPS mom Lori Walker shares in this *MOMSense* excerpt, not taking time to stoke the fires of our own creativity can make us more likely to burn out and melt down.

> As a child, I taped a sign "Writer at Work: Do not disturb!!" to my bedroom door. For hours I wrote stories . . . but, alas, everyone grows up. I had all but forgotten the pleasure I once took in writing a poem when my son Soren was born. When Soren was awake, I wanted to be with him. When he napped, I had to nap or do the laundry or pay bills or make phone calls. It didn't take very long until I felt overwhelmed and even depressed.
>
> I've learned that it's invaluable to my mothering skills that I take some time just for me. Letting my mind muse about a character I want to create or the way certain words sound just right together allows me a little escape from my practical tasks. It doesn't matter what I write, just that for a few moments, I am like Alice slipping into a Wonderland where anything is possible. And, when my son wakes from his nap, he wakes to a mom ready to engage with him in his wonderland, also a world full of creative and wonderful possibilities.[18]

What interest or passion recharges you? Is there a particular craft, hobby, or other creative outlet that you enjoy that you can bring back into your life? Or is there an activity you've always wanted to try? *You have permission to take some time for the creative side of you!* Whether it is tending a flower planted in your yard or on the window sill, creating a keepsake scrapbook, or taking up tap dancing, I'm sure you will find that engaging in even brief periods of a creative activity will lift some of the stress and anxiety from your life and enable you to be a *better* mom.

Dump out your thoughts. Another creative outlet that can dramatically decrease your stress and anxiety is what I refer to as "dumping out" your thoughts on paper. This is a little different than journaling because your goal is not to create a keepsake or even pretty prose. The goal here is to get out all the thoughts that are swirling around and creating noise in your brain. Even if all you can think to write is "I don't know what to write," or "I have to go to the grocery store," this writing can serve as a release. I learned the concept from Julia Cameron's book *The Artist's Way,* where she recommends writing out these pages every morning.[19] If evening or two minutes here or there during the day works better for you, that's fine. Just give it a try!

Give me a break! Whether you get away for ten minutes, an hour, or a day, and even if you spend the whole time talking about and thinking about your kids, a break is *still* valuable. You need and deserve breaks for refreshment! A few hours out with a girlfriend doing something enjoyable and relaxing pays off. Having a meal out that is uninterrupted by the needs of children is an amazing treat when you haven't done it for a while. Even a meal at home without kids while a friend or loved one takes the children can boost your spirits.

These ideas will get you started, but these are only the beginning. A wealth of other practical suggestions exists within these other MOPS books that will help you reduce your stress and anxiety:

- *Time Out for Busy Moms . . . Ahhh Moments* by Cynthia W. Sumner, Mary Beth Lagerborg (General Editor)
- *Juggling Tasks, Tots, and Time* by Cathy Penshorn, Mary Beth Lagerborg (General Editor)
- *Kid's Stuff and What to Do with It* by Leigh Rollar Mintz, Mary Beth Lagerborg (General Editor)
- *If You Ever Needed Friends It's Now* by Leslie Parrott, Mary Beth Lagerborg (General Editor)
- *What Every Mom Needs* by Elisa Morgan and Carol Kuykendall

The *Best* Stress and Anxiety Reduction Advice

If I had to pick only five recommendations that most effectively reduce stress, I would select the following:

1. *Physical exercise.* Directly decreases the harmful adrenaline and cortisol hormone levels and physically causes the body to relax, while doing many other healthful things in the body. It boosts energy and your mood, strengthens muscles and your heart, and even strengthens your immune system.
2. *Breathing exercises.* These directly stimulate a relaxation response in the body, leading to lower heart rate and blood pressure, muscle relaxation, and a clearer mind.
3. *Sleep.* A good night's sleep can do amazing things to restore your body and renew your mind. "Weeping may remain for a night, but rejoicing comes in the morning" (Psalm 30:5).
4. *Mind your mind.* What you think directly affects how you feel and how your physical body reacts. It is amazing how quickly a fearful or angry thought causes your heart to speed up, your blood pressure to shoot up, and your muscles to tense. What are *you* thinking? If you are struggling with a mismatch of your expectations about this whole mothering thing and the reality of what mothering really is, it is time to work through the inconsistency. Journaling, talking with friends or family, or seeking professional counseling are all smart ways to sort through your thoughts to reach a healthier perspective. But the most important thing to realize and remind yourself of is that God is always with you, in every situation, and wants to help you through everything.
5. *Seek an attitude of thankfulness, humor, and joy.* Our attitude when we are under pressure makes a huge difference in how our bodies respond to stress. Believing you are coping well, laughter itself, and practicing an attitude of thankfulness

directly decrease the harmful hormone levels of the stress response. Practicing an attitude of thankfulness means actually looking for what there is to be thankful for in any and every situation. We all face inevitable things-have-gone-wrong events, and we can cope better with the stress of these events if we have the right attitude.

But *joy* is the real key to conquering stress, anxiety, and their energy-draining effect. Joy fuels your being. Joy enables you to do whatever is necessary, even when you are bone tired. Where do you find *your* joy? When you find your joy, there, too, you will find a lot of stress and anxiety relief and a wealth of energy. Happy hunting!

3

Healthy Diet—Fueling Your Daily Mom-a-Thon

Please join me now for your personal nutrition consultation. What would our nutritionist find if you sat down with her and showed her a food diary recording *all* you ate during the last week? Are you cringing and trying to sneak out of the room? Please don't run away! We merely want to look at your typical diet in a typical week. I promise, it will just be between us.

Are you surviving on the crusts you cut off your child's grilled-cheese sandwiches? Or half-eaten peanut-butter-and-jelly sandwiches? And are you topping it off with the rest of the applesauce the baby didn't want during her noon feeding? All these bites add up as calories, but they probably aren't providing the fuel and nutrition you need.

Are you skipping meals either to try to lose weight or because you get too busy to eat? If you are, this can sabotage the rate of your metabolism, making it *slow down* and cause you to *gain weight!* Are you eliminating entire food groups because someone told you those are "bad" for you? Hopefully not because you can set yourself up for nutritional deficiencies if you exclude entire food groups.

So let's take a look at how you can keep a healthy balance in your diet by practicing moderation and being selective about your food choices—keeping *all* the food groups in your diet. Let's also ensure that you are maximizing the rate of your metabolism and eating enough calories at the right times to provide yourself with maximum energy.

Moms need real meals with *smart* calories to get them through the day. You probably never considered the I.Q. level of calories, but some seem to be smarter than others, and their intelligence often depends on what time of day you eat them. For instance, we need foods that provide maximum energy at the beginning of the day. For breakfast you need fat-containing foods and a load of carbohydrates since you have the whole day to burn these calories as fuel during your Mom-a-thon. But if you eat a high-calorie food just before bedtime, guess where it goes? It tells your body you need more padding for a good night's sleep and then migrates usually to your hips, thighs, and waist. A good general eating rule is to eat breakfast like a king, lunch like a prince, and dinner like a pauper.[1]

A Healthy Basic Plan

You have likely heard many different experts say that *theirs* is the *right* eating plan. Can they all be correct? While many of them are right, because there are important basic principles behind healthy eating plans, there is room for individual preferences beyond that. An example of this is the vegetarian approach versus the meat-eater's approach to a healthy diet. It is the *basics* behind the plans that count. A great online resource showing several of these different healthy plans—such as the Healthy Eating pyramid, the Mediterranean Diet pyramid, the Mayo Clinic pyramid, the Vegetarian pyramid, the Asian pyramid, the Adults-over-Seventy Pyramid, and the Food Guide pyramid—is www.nal.usda.gov/fnic/etext/000023.html. Other resources include the "healthy eating" website at www.usda.gov/cnpp and general information from the American Dietetic Association, at www.eatright.org.

So how do you know if your diet is healthy enough? It's likely you have a healthy diet if you

- Eat at least five to ten servings of fruits and both green and yellow vegetables per day;

- Moderately eat cereals, breads, rice, and pasta (the more whole grain varieties the better); and
- Minimize your intake of high-fat foods like red meat and cheese as well as high-sugar foods like candy.

Another plus to this approach is that families normally find that when they eat more fruits and veggies and whole grains, their food bill *decreases.*

Five important reasons to choose this type of diet:

1. May decrease breast cancer risk
2. Decreases risk of diabetes, and decreases severity of diabetes if you have it
3. Decreases coronary heart disease risk
4. Increases protection from disease because of antioxidants in fruits and vegetables
5. Supplies high energy and a stable blood sugar level

Beyond the basics, there are a lot of questions about the finer points of a healthy diet, such as, Should I eliminate carbohydrates? Should I eliminate most fat from my diet? Are certain vegetables bad for me to eat? Is it okay to eat sweets? Should I drink coffee or tea? Let's explore some of these finer points and get the scoop on eating healthy.

Fruits and Veggies Are Your Friends

A recent study found that women who were lifelong vegetarians may have a lower risk of developing breast cancer. The protective effect appears to be directly related to the quantity of vegetables and legumes consumed, not from avoiding meat. In fact, the women who ate the most veggies and legumes had up to half the risk of breast cancer as compared to those who ate the lowest quantity of these great foods.[2] How much is enough? A minimum of five servings per day is the place to start, but push your intake to come closer to ten servings per day. Why are fruits and vegetables so important? Their high-fiber content is one reason. But one of the most important reasons to gobble up these guys is that they contain high concentrations of many different disease-preventing antioxidants. For example, in addition to familiar antioxidants like beta-carotene, Vitamin C, and Vitamin A, brightly colored veggies like carrots, red bell peppers, and sweet potatoes contain a class of antioxidants called carotenoids. Broccoli, cabbage, and cauliflower contain sulforaphane and indole-3 carbinol, tomatoes have lycopene, and dark leafy veggies are rich in lutein. Citrus fruit and grapes have flavonoids, and soy foods contain isoflavones. Since each of these different antioxidants serves a different role in preventing disease, we need to eat a variety of these fruits and veggies to get the best protection from disease in general. As in the study above, a multitude of research studies connect eating the antioxidants in fruit and vegetable form with lower rates of cancer, heart disease, diabetes, and many other diseases. At this time, research has *not* found the same great results when antioxidants are taken isolated as nutritional supplements. Many studies do show that antioxidant supplements are beneficial. But you are wise to increase the fruits and vegetables in your diet rather than depending solely on a daily antioxidant pill and hoping for the same results.

Fresh, Frozen, or Canned?

Which form of fruits and especially veggies is healthier—fresh, frozen, or canned? It may surprise you to learn that often frozen fruits and veggies have more nutritional value than fresh produce! It depends how long the fresh variety has been around and what conditions it was subjected to en route from field to fridge. One example to keep in mind concerns ready-to-drink versus frozen orange juice. A recent university study found that a cup of frozen reconstituted OJ had *twice* the vitamin C as a cup from a just opened carton of ready-to-drink OJ! This study also measured the vitamin C content of each type as time went by (in the fridge). In both the ready-to-drink and the frozen OJ, as time went, so did the vitamin C. In fact, by four weeks after opening the carton, many cartons of the ready-to-drink OJ had *zero* vitamin C, and the frozen OJ had about half as much vitamin C per serving. So the moral of this story is: consider going back to frozen reconstituted OJ if you thought the "fresh" kind was healthier, and if you prefer to stick with the ready-to-drink type, then try to drink it within a week after opening.[3]

Are Potatoes and Carrots "Bad" for You?

Certain weight-loss plans claim it is wrong to eat vegetables like potatoes and carrots since they raise the blood sugar too quickly and stimulate more insulin to be released than other vegetables do. This action on the bloodstream by food items is commonly referred to as the "glycemic index," with a high glycemic index meaning that a food raises the blood sugar rapidly and to a high level. If you eat these veggies as part of a meal, I have no concern. When you eat high glycemic foods along with protein and complex carbohydrates, there is not the same dramatic effect on the blood sugar and insulin levels. Don't abandon these starchy veggies, for they are packed with important nutrients. I will not have us eliminating healthy foods from our diets if I can help it!

Carbohydrates Are Not the Enemy

Carbohydrates have been getting a bad rap lately. This is partly due to certain high-protein-high-fat diet plans that claim this food group is the enemy and should be avoided. However, carbohydrates are the foods that *most affect your energy level.* They should not be eliminated from your diet; rather, they should be used wisely. The good carbs I am referring to are complex carbohydrates—whole grain bread, whole grain cereal, brown rice, bulgur, oats, legumes, and many other grains and vegetables. Complex carbohydrates are filling, release energy to you slowly and steadily as they are digested, and are high in fiber too.

When I need an energy boost or I'm hungry between meals, I have a satisfying serving of brown rice or other whole grains. But these foods take time to cook, so every few days I cook several cups of grains in my rice cooker and store the surplus in the fridge. Then I can grab a quick serving, heat it for thirty seconds in the microwave, and eat it whenever I need it. When it comes to simple carbohydrates like pasta, bread, and cereal not made of whole grains, and sugary foods, the real issue is what quantity you eat and how many total calories you take in. These foods do not automatically make you gain weight. It is the quantity that's the culprit.

If you need another good reason to eat carbohydrates, I have one for all stressed moms out there. "Comfort food" carbohydrates may actually help you biochemically to handle stress in a less damaging way. According to Mary F. Dallman, University of California San Francisco researcher and professor of physiology, separate studies with both rats and humans show that those who ate lots of carbohydrates prior to being subjected to very stressful tasks actually released *less* cortisol (one of the stress hormones) and had less depression after the experiment was completed.[4]

Protein—Don't Leave a Meal without It

Protein is important to eat at every meal because it contains the building blocks of our muscles and helps stabilize the blood sugar level. But we need to be aware of the type and total amount of protein that we eat daily. To be most healthy, any type of animal protein should be lean, without any visible fat. A good rule of thumb (or should I say "rule of palm") is to choose a serving-size portion of meat that is roughly the size of your palm. If eating chicken, it's healthiest to remove the skin before cooking (that's where most of the fat is) or at least before eating.

How much protein should you eat in a day? The recommended daily allowance (RDA) is a third of a gram for every pound of your body weight. The calculation is 0.36 x your weight in pounds = quantity of protein needed per day, in grams (grams/day). To put that in perspective, that's about 50 grams per day for a woman weighing 140 pounds. Most adults in this country easily meet this daily requirement. In fact, many exceed it substantially. Too much protein in your diet can be hard on both your kidneys and liver. So if you load up on protein, be certain to drink lots of water to help flush out the body and protect your kidneys.

Here is a rough guide to how much protein is in your entrée:

- *Lean meat or poultry* 6 oz. = 50 grams protein
- *Fish* 6 oz. = 40 grams

- *Eggs* 2 large = 12 grams
- *Milk or yogurt* 1 cup = 8 grams
- *Cheese* 1 oz. = 6–8 grams
- *Peanut butter* 2 tablespoons = 8 grams
- *Soybeans* (see below)

Soybeans and Other Beans and Nuts

You've heard a lot more about beans and nuts in recent years because they are highly nutritious, excellent sources of protein; yes, we are talking about none other than soybeans and other legumes like pintos, chickpeas, navy beans, and lentils, and certain friends in the nut family. Soy foods are highly acclaimed now because in 2000, based on over fifty studies, the FDA concluded that eating 25 grams of soy protein a day as part of a healthy diet could help reduce the risk of heart disease and lower cholesterol. Many studies confirmed that it is the combination of soy protein and isoflavones (another component of soy) that leads to a decrease in cholesterol levels and other healthy heart changes. Either soy protein or isoflavones alone do not yield the same helpful results. Don't be deceived into buying soy supplements on the market that contain only isoflavones. Eat whole soy foods instead. Soy foods also help many women cope better with the physical symptoms of menopause. We will look at these benefits further in chapter 16.

Great common sources of soy protein and isoflavones include:[5]

- *Edamame* (whole soybeans in pods, you steam or boil) 3/4 cup shelled = 25 grams soy protein
- *Roasted soybeans* 1 cup roasted = 25 grams soy protein
- *Soy flour* 1/4 cup = 47 grams
- *Soy milk* 1 cup = 13 grams
- *Tofu* (firm) 4 ounces = 13 grams, or (soft) 4 ounces = 9 grams
- *Tempeh* 4 ounces = 17 grams

50 Ways to Get Your Soy

With all these great reasons to use soy foods, consider adding them to your weekly meals and snacks. If you aren't familiar with soybean food products, and your only previous experience with soy is "soy sauce" (*not* a nutritious form of soy), take heart! There are many easy ways to learn how to use them. Edamame (in most grocers' freezer vegetable sections) is a great way to begin to use soy. Just put these frozen pods in a bowl, cover with water, and microwave for about five minutes. Then rinse with cool water, drain, and eat. Pop them right out of the pod into your mouth (or dish if you wish). Kids love them. (But don't give them to very young children, who could choke on them.) Another great snack idea is to buy roasted soy nuts to munch on instead of other nuts. They are available plain, salted, and with seasonings such as barbeque. Again, beware that these, like peanuts, are a choking hazard for young children.

If you like fruit smoothies, consider substituting soy milk in place of cow's milk. Or try a flavored soy milk as your beverage. Although many people agree that soy milk by itself is not the best-tasting way to get soy, Consumer Reports rated Vitasoy Vanilla Delite and Silk Vanilla as very good tasting soy milk and Soy Dream Vanilla Enriched and Sun Soy Vanilla as good tasting.[6] Soy drink products I like are the Revival brand soy drink mixes (available directly from the company: 1-800-500-2055, www.revivalsoy.com). The chocolate tastes as good as Nestle's Quik! They also have flavors such as vanilla, strawberry, peach, and even cappuccino. One serving of this mix delivers 20 grams of soy protein. Most soy drink mixes are hard to recommend for they are not made from whole soybeans, but all of Revival's products are real soy food. Revival also makes several flavors of soy crisp bars (that are like Rice Krispie treats—only healthy) that are delicious and deliver 17 grams of protein per bar. Both the drink mixes and bars make great meal replacements. Revival also sells delicious soy nuts covered with real chocolate for snacking, in addition to many other flavors of roasted soy nuts.

Tofu is very mild in taste, which means it is an easy way to add soy to some of your favorite recipes, for it picks up the flavors of other items.

Try adding diced pieces of tofu to your spaghetti sauce, soups, stews, and other entrees. I recommend a great tofu cookbook, *This Can't Be Tofu!* by Deborah Madison. In it she instructs how to use different kinds of tofu to create everything from "Smoked Tofu with Barbeque Sauce" to "Curried 'Chicken' Salad." She also hides tofu in the sauce in recipes such as "Poached Salmon and Potatoes with Fresh Herb Sauce."[7] A wonderful free website with a wide range of soy food recipes is the U.S. Soyfoods Directory site's "Soyfood Cookbook" at www.soyfood.com. In the vast selection you are sure to find several recipes that you and your family will enjoy. The iVillage free website offers nearly forty recipes from *The Whole Soy Cookbook,* such as "Soy Pancakes" and "Applesauce Cake," which may be a sweet way to work soy into your diet (www.ivillage.com/food/hltheat/specfood/articles/0,11731,165797_6074,00.html).

Experiment with adding different forms of soy to your diet. There will likely be some forms you like and some you could live without, but you have little to lose and lots of nutrition and health benefits to gain.

Not All Fats Are Created Equal

With all the focus lately on how bad fat is for us, have you started to wonder if you should cut it out all together? Actually, this would be a *bad* idea. Some types of fat are so essential to our health that they are called "*essential* fats." But there are definitely good and bad types in the fat clan, so let's meet them so you know who to invite into your diet and who to limit your exposure to. Two points to remember about fats include the following:

1. Fats from vegetable sources are generally better for you than fats from animal sources, although there are some exceptions to that rule.
2. Fats in liquid form at room temperature are generally better for you than those that are in a more solid form at room temperature.

The "Good Guys" of the Fat Clan

The good fats include the essential fatty acids and fats as well as monounsaturated and polyunsaturated fats. You need a certain amount of these good fats for healthy brain function (structural components in your brain are made from fats we consume) and to have enough of the good HDL form of cholesterol. The essential fats (including omega-3 and omega-6 fats) are called "essential" because they are crucial to good health, yet the body cannot make them. They must come from food or supplements. The omega-3 fats are very important to heart health. Studies show they reduce triglyceride levels and bad LDL cholesterol levels in the blood, reduce the stickiness of platelets, and help to prevent clots that cause heart attacks. These omega-3 fats can also prevent abnormal heart rhythms that lead to cardiac arrest.[8] Great sources for omega-3 fats are fatty fish like tuna, salmon, mackerel, and sardines, plus flaxseeds, walnuts, and soy beans.

The biggest surprise in this group is peanuts. Eating peanuts or peanut butter may actually *decrease* your overall cholesterol level while also increasing your good HDL cholesterol, because peanuts are rich in monounsaturated fat. There is strong evidence that eating the right kinds of fats—namely monounsaturated and polyunsaturated fats—may actually *decrease* your incidence of heart disease. These fats are the main reason the American Heart Association recently revised its policy on fats. The AHA now recommends that a heart-healthy diet can have up to 35 to 40 percent of daily calories from fat, a substantial jump from the previous rule of only 30 percent of daily calories coming from fat. The fact that we need a sensible amount of good fat in our diets was confirmed by a recent study in which a diet very low in fat was found to be *less* heart healthy than a diet with a lot of monounsaturated fats![9] Peanuts, unprocessed peanut butter, and peanut oil are excellent sources for monounsaturated fats, as are olive oil, canola oil, and avocados.[10]

Although peanut butter is good for you, it is important to choose unprocessed brands instead of those with lots of sugar and saturated fat. Most grocery stores carry Laura Scudder's "All Natural Old-Fashioned

Peanut Butter." If you check the labels, you probably will find other unprocessed brands at your grocers. You should easily find unprocessed peanut butter in health food stores. You will note that this type of peanut butter often "settles out" a layer of oil on top with thick peanut goo below. But if you stir it well and refrigerate it, it will look like regular crunchy peanut butter. If you were used to Jif and Skippy and other processed brands, you'll have to adjust to the less sugary taste of Laura Scudder's and other brands that are good for you. They really are tasty and the switch is powerfully good for the health of everyone in your family. Just think of all the peanut butter sandwiches your children will eat in their lifetime. Isn't it a good idea to get them hooked on a healthy kind now?

The "Bad Guys" of the Fat Clan

The bad fats include saturated fats that come from animal sources (which are known to increase cholesterol, especially the bad LDL cholesterol), and trans fats used to stabilize store-bought foods like crackers and baked goods. Trans fats, which started out as a good unsaturated fat, may now be the worst fat around. In food-processing plants this unsaturated fat is converted to a partially hydrogenated fat. This stabilizes store-bought products so they last longer. These trans fats are now known to be the worst culprit for causing clogging in the arteries. They also increase the bad LDL level in the blood and decrease the good HDL cholesterol levels.

The Dish on Fish

Fish is high in protein, low in bad fats, high in important and healthy omega-3 fats—what's not to love? Well, the truth is, some of you don't love the taste of fish. In that case, get flaxseeds from your local health food store and either grind them up or buy them already ground (they will last four months in the refrigerator), then sprinkle about 1 to 2 tablespoons on your food each day. Or, if you prefer, take 1 tablespoon of flaxseed oil daily. This gives you the same omega-3 fatty acids without

Know Your Fats Table Info from the American Heart Association

FAT	SOURCE	RISKS and BENEFITS
Saturated Fats	Meat, Tropical oils, Dairy	The main dietary culprit in raising blood cholesterol
"Trans Fats" Hydrogenated fat (Produced by a chemical process that changes a liquid oil to a more solid and saturated form)	Commercial products like crackers, chips, cookies (look for hydrogenated or partially hydrogenated fat on ingredient list)	Many studies suggest that these fats raise blood total cholesterol and LDL (bad) cholesterol, and lower HDL (good) cholesterol
Monounsaturated Fats	Canola, Olive, and Peanut oil, Avocado	May lower your blood cholesterol
Polyunsaturated Fats	Safflower, sesame, and sunflower seeds; corn and soybeans; many other nuts, seeds, and their oils; and fatty fish	May help your body get rid of newly formed cholesterol and may lower cholesterol level when used in place of saturated fats in your diet

eating something fishy. But, if possible, eat the recommended two to three 3-ounce servings a week of cold-water fatty fish such as tuna, salmon, or mackerel. Pregnant and nursing women need to be concerned about the potential for significant mercury contamination in certain fish, so they must avoid fresh tuna, shark, swordfish, king mackerel, and tilefish, plus limit canned tuna to 5 ounces per week.[11]

Strengthen Your Constitution with Fiber

Fiber helps your health in numerous ways. Fiber may lower your risk of heart disease and diabetes. It lowers your cholesterol, speeds food through your digestive tract to keep your bowels functioning well, possibly protects against colon cancer, and gives you a feeling of fullness, which discourages you from overeating.[12] The protection against colon cancer does not appear to be strong if we get most of our fiber from supplements available in drug stores. Research shows that the connection is strongest when the fiber grams come from whole foods rich in fiber—which means eating lots of veggies and fruits.

The average American intake is 10 to 15 grams of fiber per day, which is very low, considering the Surgeon General and the National Cancer Institute recommend 20 to 35 grams per day. That means most of us need to be looking for ways to increase the fiber in our diets. *Soluble* fiber (pectin) is found in apples, pears, and oats; it mops up the inside of the intestine and, among other things, traps cholesterol. *Insoluble* fiber, often called "roughage," is found in vegetables like celery and other coarse whole grains. Two words of caution about increasing fiber in your diet: *add slowly.* Otherwise you will wonder if this health benefit is worth the discomfort, gas, and bloating.

Do You Eat Enough Fiber?

How does your dietary fiber add up? Here are some guidelines from the American Institute for Cancer Research:

"A serving of fruits or vegetables is equal to just one apple or peach, one-half cup of pineapple chunks, one-half cup of chopped broccoli or one-quarter cup of raisins. Servings of grains and beans add up even faster. The two slices of bread on a sandwich equal two servings, as does a cup of rice or pasta. A cup of beans equals two servings, and you can wrap them in a whole-wheat tortilla for one more. Your morning bowl of cereal probably contains two or more servings." Now, using this chart, add it all up to see if you meet your daily fiber requirement of 20 to 35 grams of fiber per day.

Figure out how much fiber you eat in a day:

Number of daily servings		Fiber per serving (gms)	Total (grams)
____	Beans, lentils	x 6	= ____
____	Fruits, vegetables, whole grains, nuts	x 2.5	= ____
____	Refined grains (white bread, white rice, regular pasta)	x 1	= ____
____	Other grains (including breakfast cereals)	x (ck label)	= ____
	Total grams of dietary fiber		= ____

Source: American Institute for Cancer Research, *The Facts about Fiber* (brochure), 2001. Available online or to order at www.airc.org/index.lasso.

What Is the Fiber Content in My Food?

Ever wonder about the fiber content in jelly beans? (It's zero, by the way.) Just about any food you can think of is ranked by fiber content in the U.S. Department of Agriculture's resource "USDA Nutrient Database for Standard Reference, Release 15" (ranks more than a thousand foods) at www.nal.usda.gov/fnic/foodcomp/Data/SR15/wtrank/st15a291.pdf. Or you can see the same foods and fiber content listed alphabetically at www.nal.usda.gov/fniv/foodcomp/Data/SR15/wtrank/sr15a291.pdf.

Here's a handy table that lists many common high-fiber foods. Do any of these surprise you?

How Will You Get Your Fill of Fiber?

If you are like most people, you probably need to add more fiber to your diet. Let's find ways to add fiber that work specifically for you. You can take the "add one mega-fiber food to my diet" approach, and eat a one-cup serving of General Mills' Fiber One cereal—which would deliver 28 grams of fiber, or one cup of Kellogg's All-Bran, which will give you 20 grams of fiber per serving. Another easy way to add fiber is the "substitution way," which means you look for any chance to substitute a higher fiber alternative to what you would normally eat. For instance, eat pieces of fruit instead of drinking juice. Substitute whole grain brown rice, Kashi, or bulgur anytime you would usually eat white rice. Stick with whole grain breads instead of processed, white-type breads. (You can tell they are whole grain if a whole grain is listed as the first ingredient on the label.)

Then there is the "add a little to every meal" way of adding additional servings of fresh fruits and vegetables to each meal or as snacks. They add up. Or perhaps you'd prefer to "sprinkle it on throughout the day" by sprinkling miller's bran or ground flaxseed meal onto foods, such as cereal, yogurt, or fruit and even soups and casseroles. Miller's bran is pure bran (found in health food stores) and brings a whopping dose of fiber per teaspoon. You can also add miller's bran to any recipe for bread, muffins, or pancakes. Flaxseed meal delivers 4 grams of fiber

High-Fiber Foods

Food	Serving Size	Amount of Fiber in grams (g)
Vegetables		
Potato, baked with skin	1 medium	5
Acorn squash, baked	½ cup	5
Mixed vegetables, frozen	½ cup	4
Carrots	½ cup	3
Broccoli	½ cup	2
Corn kernels	½ cup	2
Spinach, raw	1 cup	1
Fruit		
Apple, with skin	1 medium	4
Blueberries	½ cup	4
Apricots, dried	¼ cup	3
Banana	1 medium	3
Orange	1 medium	3
Strawberries	½ cup	2
Grapefruit	½ large	2
Legumes		
Lentils	½ cup, cooked	8
Split peas	½ cup, cooked	8
Kidney beans, black beans	½ cup, cooked	7
Hummus	½ cup	6
Grains/Breads		
Bulgur	½ cup, cooked	4
Whole wheat spaghetti	½ cup, cooked	3
Barley	½ cup, cooked	3
Whole wheat pita	½ pita (6 ½")	3
Brown rice	½ cup, cooked	2
Whole wheat bread	1 slice	2
Enriched spaghetti	½ cup, cooked	1
Bagel, plain	bagel (3 ½")	1
White rice, instant long-grain	½ cup, cooked	1
White bread	1 slice	1

Source: U.S. Department of Agriculture

American Institute for Cancer Research. 2001. The Facts about Fiber (brochure).

in every 2 tablespoons in addition to the omega-3 and omega-6 fatty acids. If none of these options will work for you, you can add a daily fiber supplement, such as bran tablets (health food store), or a drinkable form of fiber like Metamucil, FiberCon, or FiberWise. Most of these products deliver about 4 grams of fiber per serving. Or eat a high-fiber bar like FiberWise bars, with 3.5 grams per serving;[14] but beware. Check labels. Some so-called "fiber bars" actually contain very little fiber! For example, Nutri-grain bars are tasty but have only 1 gram of fiber (and up to 15 grams of sugar) per bar.

Here's a motivating tidbit about fiber: For every gram of fiber you eat, it's estimated you can subtract about 9 calories from those you took in that day. Fiber speeds the food along through your digestive tract before all of it can be absorbed and stored as fat. Nine calories does not sound like much, but if you eat the recommended 20 to 30 grams of fiber each day, that's 180 to 270 calories you get to subtract from your total calorie intake, and that can be a great help if you are working to lose weight.

Calcium—A Vital Force in Women's Nutrition

Calcium does many things that are crucial to the functioning of a woman's body. It takes part in countless cell reactions day in and day out, has a role in stabilizing blood pressure, decreases PMS, and, of course, helps prevent osteoporosis. Sixty percent of women ages sixty-five to seventy-four have low bone mass, and 20 percent have osteoporosis. By age seventy-five, 35 percent of women have osteoporosis, and by age eighty-five, more than 50 percent of women have osteoporosis.[15] The catch is your body cannot manufacture calcium; it must come from outside your body. We use and lose calcium every day, so it must be replaced regularly. And calcium can be difficult to absorb even if you take in enough.

How much calcium is enough? It depends on your age. Women in general are advised to take in 1,000 mg of calcium a day. At age fifty this should increase to 1,200 to 1,500 mg a day, and at age sixty-five, 1,500 mg a day. Although osteoporosis is not usually evident until after menopause, you need to tank up your bones throughout your preadult and young adult years so that you start out menopause with the best chance of holding on to your bone mass.

The best food sources for calcium include:[16]

- Plain nonfat yogurt = 450 mg/cup
- Fruit yogurt = 300 mg/cup
- Milk = 300 mg/cup
- Calcium-fortified orange juice = 300 mg/cup
- Swiss cheese = 270 mg/1 oz.
- Pizza = 250 mg/4 oz. slice
- Salmon = 225 mg/3 oz.
- Cheddar cheese = 200 mg/1 oz.
- Cooked turnip greens = 200 mg/cup
- Soybeans = 130 mg/ 1/2 cup
- Cooked broccoli = 90 mg/cup

Most women do not take in enough calcium through their foods, so they need a calcium supplement. You should not take more than a 500 mg supplement at a time, for that is the most the body can absorb at a sitting. Furthermore, calcium is best absorbed when surrounded by its "buddies": 400 to 800 IU vitamin D, and 400 mg magnesium.

Get Your Daily Dose of Beneficial Bacteria

It may be odd to imagine that we would *want* to put bacteria into our bodies for better health, but there are beneficial bacteria you want to have around, such as lactobacillus. These good bacteria populate your gastrointestinal and vaginal tracts and protect you from an overgrowth of harmful bacteria or yeast. Eating at least one serving a day of yogurt is a wise way to get calcium and these good bacteria. Just make sure the brand you buy says "Live and Active Culture Yogurt" on the label.

When There Isn't Time for a Real Meal

You still need to eat, even when there isn't time. Make time for a fast and easy meal. Try a drinkable yogurt along with a portable piece of fruit, or an ultra-quick peanut butter sandwich, or string cheese wrapped in a piece of bread and served with a piece of fruit. Some of the food and meal bars on the market are worth considering, as are some of the meal replacement drink products (which we will discuss further in chapter 5). But nutrition gaps widen if you depend on these regularly for too much of your daily sustenance.

Ideally, you want to have all your food groups at each meal, but let's be practical. If the choice comes down to not eating at all (or having only a few leftover sandwich crusts), then meal replacement products are a good alternative. Look at the label and avoid those that have corn syrup solids or sucrose as the first ingredient, which means the product is packed with refined sugar. Fructose, the sugar from fruit, is a better sugar source. Also look for either soy protein or whey for the main protein source in meal replacement products. Again, a good meal replacement solution is Revival brand soy drink mix or bars.[17]

> *"My problem is that either I snack all day long or I forget to eat."*
>
> *—Patricia*

Where Sweets Fit

In an ideal world we would not have cravings for fudge brownies or Häagen-Dazs ice cream (although I personally hope we can still get these in heaven). Here in the real world, we do. Since it is difficult to turn your back completely on sweets, let's at least find the healthiest ways to eat them.

For starters, one of the worst times to eat candy, cookies, and the like is when you have an empty stomach. The goodies send a big load of simple sugar and fat rushing into your bloodstream, which doesn't make your body very happy. Because of the big load of sugar, your pancreas sends out an equally big load of insulin to counteract the high level of sugar. This process works, but maybe a little too well, because the next thing you know, your blood sugar level plummets, often leaving you with an even lower blood sugar level than you had before you ate the sweet snack.

A better way to eat sweets is right after a substantial meal. This way the rise in your blood sugar isn't as strong since your body has already sent out insulin to handle the other food you've eaten. And afterward your blood sugar level doesn't fall so dramatically either. It is especially important that the meal have a serving of protein—or at the very least, have a glass of milk before the sweets. The protein makes a big difference in stabilizing your blood sugar level.

The Healthiest Sweets

The issue of which sweets are the healthiest is a tough one, because experts have differing opinions. It is safe to say that sweets with the least amount of added simple sugar are better. This means that desserts using fruit and deriving their sweetness mainly from the fruit are healthier than those with lots of sugar. Ice cream has the redeeming feature that it contains some calcium in every serving, but you need to watch out for the saturated fat content in the scoop of your choice. There are so many different ice cream–like products available, from sorbets to reduced-fat ice cream and the old standby, sherbet. Check out the nutritional facts on the label for the *real* scoop on these alternatives to ice cream.

Chocolate, especially dark chocolate, is getting many rave reviews because studies show it contains high levels of natural antioxidants.[18] One well-done study found that cocoa may decrease LDL (bad) cholesterol and raise HDL (good) cholesterol, both of which can decrease heart disease.[19] But chocolate also contains certain fats that are not the healthiest, so eat in moderation if chocolate is your sweet-of-choice. Remember that the trans fatty acids in many store-bought bakery goods and the saturated fats in items made with lots of butter need to be limited, because both types are the fats most likely to contribute to the clogging of your arteries.

Have I taken the fun out of your daily doughnut fix? Just remember that the sweet things in life do not *all* have loads of sucrose, trans fatty acids, and saturated fats, and even the ones that do are okay to eat on a *limited* basis!

Water Your Body

You've seen what a lack of watering does to your plants, haven't you? Well, your limbs won't exactly wilt and shrivel, but the cells of your body don't like being dehydrated. The strange thing about your thirst mechanism is that it doesn't clue you in to the amount of water you really need because it turns on too late and turns off too early. When you feel thirsty, you may already be short by up to six glasses, but it is likely you will feel refreshed after drinking only a cup or two. Some water-wise rules of thumb are:

1. Drink at least six to seven glasses of water or other beverage every day—the experts have decreased the daily requirement from eight glasses after several hydration studies found no evidence to support the "eight-a-day" rule.[20] To help you get in the habit of drinking, keep a sports bottle full where you will see it. Then drink a little frequently.
2. Six glasses per day is the *minimum* for *normal* conditions. If the weather is hot, you are perspiring a lot, or are ill and losing fluids, you need to increase the fluids you drink.
3. When you are thirsty, figure you need several glasses of fluid just to catch up.
4. Clean, clear water is the best choice, but studies show that other beverages *do count* toward your daily quota, and that even caffeinated beverages work well to hydrate.[21]

Tea—The Brew That Enhances Your Health

Whether your preference is black tea, green tea, or oolong tea, you've made a healthy choice when you brew a couple cups each day. In fact, studies show that these teas might be even healthier for you than most herbal teas, and even more protective of your health than many fruits and vegetables![22] Just like the healthy effects of fruits and vegetables, these three types of tea are chock full of the strong polyphenol flavonoid antioxidants.

These antioxidants are believed to protect our cells from damage. Studies suggest that drinking several cups of freshly brewed tea each day can protect against cancers of the lung, stomach, esophagus, colon, breast, pancreas, and liver, although we still need more research to know for sure.[23] There is also strong evidence that drinking two cups a day is very protective for your heart and may help reduce the risk of heart attack by up to 50 percent. Tea may also beef up your bones. Studies in Britain found that older female black-tea drinkers had 5 percent greater bone density than those who did not drink tea.[24] So feel free to brew your tea, and enjoy all the good it's doing for you!

Caffeine and Coffee—Comrades in Crime?

Often coffee and caffeine are blamed for a multitude of crimes, but it can be difficult to determine whether it is coffee or caffeine that is causing health issues. In general, coffee is fine if taken in moderation (two cups a day). Recent research has cleared coffee of many bad raps. For instance, coffee made through a filter in the "American-way" was *not* shown to increase blood cholesterol levels, unlike coffee made the "European way" without filters.[25]

Coffee has also been cleared of many charges about its effect on pregnant moms and their fetuses. Studies show no increase in the risk of miscarriage or low birth weight unless Mom consumes huge amounts of coffee each day (more than five cups daily). The official recommendation is for pregnant women to limit their intake to one to two cups per day.[26]

Word from other studies suggests coffee may be a "good-doer"—or is it the caffeine? One respected study showed that those who did not drink coffee were two to three times more likely to develop Parkinson's disease than those who drank one to four cups of coffee a day. However, caffeine was identified as the protective substance.[27] Another study suggests that those who drink two to three cups of coffee per day cut their risk of gallstones by 40 percent.[28] After a recent analysis of seventeen studies, coffee has also been dubbed as having a protective effect against colon cancer—there was a 24 percent lower risk for those who drink four or more cups a day.[29] Coffee may soon be thought to be heart-healthy because coffee beans, like tea, also contain high amounts of the antioxidants polyphenols, which future studies may confirm are protective for the heart and cells of the body.

Clearly, caffeine is a controversial substance in drinks and foods. Many use it because it makes us alert, may improve our concentration, and often gives us more energy, motivation, and a sense of well-being or "a lift." Others avoid caffeine because it is a stimulant and, historically, has been given a bad reputation. The truth is there are fewer proven problems from caffeine than you might think. Studies show that caffeine may cause heart palpitations, insomnia, and anxiety, and we know it is habit-forming and can cause withdrawal headaches. Increased spinal bone loss has been linked to older women's caffeine intake of 300 mg or more a day (about 3 cups of coffee), but not for younger women.[30]

Whichever side of the caffeine fence you choose, you need to know how much caffeine you are getting. The actual caffeine content of some drinks and foods may surprise you. Some, like chocolate and hot cocoa, stand with decaf coffee on the low end of the caffeine scale (5–10 mgs per serving). Black tea, green tea, Coca-Cola, and a 1-ounce shot of espresso all have about the same moderate amount of caffeine (30–50 mgs per serving). Brewed coffee is the "caffeine king," often with more caffeine in 1 cup than in 4 cans of Coca-Cola (85–175 mg per cup)! Also be aware that certain brands of root beer and orange soda (especially Sunkist) have substantial caffeine.[31] This might explain why your preschooler was wide awake at bedtime the last time she had Sunkist soda!

Why We Eat

Do you *eat to live* or *live to eat?* British author Henry Fielding suggests we do both.[32] Eating is a God-given pleasure, but it serves a much more important purpose than just enjoyment. For the energy you need to live your busy life, you need proper fuel and nutrients throughout your day. There should be no skipping of meals and no eliminating of major food groups, especially carbohydrates. Your body, to work optimally, needs the full balance of nutrients. One of the best ways to improve your health is to make wise nutrition choices. Practice what you learned in this chapter and you will have more energy, from the right sources!

Although the best way to get all your nutrients is directly from food, many moms need nutritional supplements to fill in their nutritional gaps. Let's go now to the next chapter for information on supplements that fill these gaps and may boost your energy.

4

Boosting Your Energy with Nutritional Supplements

Wouldn't it be great if we could just pop a nutritional supplement in our mouths every time we needed more energy? Magically we would have all the energy we needed, whenever we needed it, with no side effects. I'm sure you've already figured out that it's not that simple. And anyone who tells you that nutritional supplements provide everything you need is misinformed.

Nutritional supplements are just what they say they are—they *supplement* your diet to *improve* your nutrition. Supplements *do not* replace food. Even the wisest biochemists and researchers have not yet figured out all that makes food tick, so depending on supplements for the bulk of your nutrition can leave you with gaps in your nutrition.

That said, I am not one of those doctors who believes all supplements are worthless. In fact, I *strongly support* the use of nutritional supplements. But you need to take the right ones, in the right amounts, at the right times, and for the right reasons. Furthermore, all these "rights" need to be supported by reliable research.

"What vitamins should I be taking?"

Vitamins and Minerals Are Required

The "right ones" start with a balanced vitamin and mineral supplement. "Balanced" because your body needs the full spectrum of vitamins and minerals. You need excellent nutrition for your body to work optimally, and you need your body to work optimally if you want to have maximum energy. Many of us do not get all the nutrients we need, especially the vitamins and minerals, in the food we eat. Vitamins and minerals are essential for nearly all the processes in the body to run properly and efficiently. When any of these vital components are low in quantity, your body cannot function optimally, which in turn can make you feel and function poorly. Another reason supporting the need for these supplements is that the body cannot produce all the vitamins you need, and it doesn't produce *any* of the minerals! You have to get all of them from what you eat or drink—or through a nutritional supplement.

The medical community recently took a big step forward when the American Medical Association (AMA) issued a formal endorsement recommending the daily use of a basic multivitamin supplement for all adults. According to their research, "most people do not consume an optimal amount of all vitamins by diet alone."[1] They took this stand after reviewing thirty years of studies confirming that suboptimal levels of vitamins are associated with increased risk of chronic diseases such as cancer, osteoporosis, and cardiovascular disease.[2] For example, studies have shown that B vitamins folate, B-6, and B-12 decrease homocysteine levels, which results in less coronary heart disease. Increased folic acid levels in pregnant women prevent neural tube defects (spina bifida) in infants; decreases in bone loss and fractures occur if calcium and vitamin D supplements are taken together. This AMA recommendation is a very big step because, until recently, all doctors were taught that if one eats a reasonable diet, one does not need to take vitamin supplements. Doctors also believed that unless there were distinct signs of a vitamin or mineral deficiency, taking vitamins and minerals would not help one's health. You've come a long way, Doc!

The Right Vitamin and Mineral Supplement for You

In 1999, nearly half of all American adults were taking vitamins, while one-quarter of all adults were taking herbal supplements.[3] The cost of all this was an estimated $14 billion per year spent on vitamins, minerals, and herbal products.[4] But which supplements are right for you? If you are pregnant, nursing, or trying to get pregnant, be sure to take the supplement prescribed by your physician, because at these times women need at least 400 mcg per day of folic acid (or folate). Women also need more calcium, but need to be careful not to take too much Vitamin A (should not exceed 10,000 units per day).

Basic Model or Mega Model?

The rest of us have to make a decision—whether to go with the *basic model* or the *mega model* vitamin and mineral supplement. The general recommendation is that we take a balanced, multivitamin/multimineral supplement that contains the RDAs, or recommended daily allowances, of these nutrients. This is what I term the basic model, because the RDA is the minimum amount of that nutrient required each day.

But what about those vitamin and mineral supplements that contain *more than* the RDA of many nutrients? These supplements are formulated on the principle that taking higher-than-the-RDA amounts of certain nutrients may be even more helpful in preventing certain degenerative diseases. In addition, many of us require a lot more than the RDA of certain nutrients, such as when we are stressed, ill, exposed to a toxic environment, or getting older, one of which probably covers the majority of us. Research studies support the above-RDA quantities of many of these nutrients, but there are not yet enough studies for the AMA to endorse megadoses of these nutrients.

Safe Upper Limits

However, we do have a list of the "upper intake levels" for different vitamins and minerals. This information came out of testing done by the Food and Nutrition Board (the same ones who establish the RDA values) and the National Academy of Sciences. The table below lists the upper intake levels for some of the more common nutrients. What do these upper limits mean? This is the level at which we might begin to see an adverse effect on the body. This is approaching a "danger" level, but still not high enough to be considered truly dangerous. Choosing multivitamin and multimineral supplements with nutrient quantities less than or equal to the upper limits should be safe.

Safe Upper Limits for Common Vitamins and Minerals[5]		
Nutrient	**Daily Value**	**Upper Intake Levels**
Vitamin A (retinol)	5,000 IU (or mcg)	10,000 IU (or mcg)
Beta-carotene	5,000 IU (if instead of retinol)	none set–nontoxic
Niacin (Vit. B-3)	20 mg	35 mg
Vitamin B-6	2 mg	100 mg
Vitamin B-12	6 mcg	non set
Folate (Folic Acid)	400 mcg	1,000 mcg or 1 gram
Vitamin C	90 mg	2,000 mg
Vitamin D	400 IU	2,000 IU
Vitamin E	22 IU natural or	1,500 IU natural or
Vitamin E	30 IU synthetic	1,100 IU synthetic

Vitamin K	80 mcg	none set
Calcium	1,000 mg (1,200 if > age 50)	2,500 mg
Magnesium	320 mg	350 mg
Phosphorus	1,000 mg	4,000 mg
Iron	18 mg	45 mg
Zinc	15 mg	40 mg
Chromium	120 mcg	none set
Copper	2 mg	10 mg
Selenium	70 mcg	400 mcg

What Will You Spend?

Another factor in deciding which is the right supplement for you is determining how much you are willing to spend. The range is very wide, from a few dollars a month to as high as $70 to $100 per month. Why the broad range? The moderate-to-higher priced product suppliers justify the price by ensuring the highest quality ingredients, formulas based on the latest research, testing of products for purity and potency, and may also say disintegration tests prove the product will dissolve properly so it can be absorbed in the body. Many customers of these moderate-to-higher-priced supplements claim they "feel the difference" between not feeling energetic when they were on a basic model supplement and feeling much more energy on a mega model supplement.

Don't Buy à la Carte

Many women buy their vitamins and minerals the à la carte way, choosing a bottle of vitamin C here, a bottle of calcium there. I don't recommend this approach. Vitamins and minerals work in concert to maintain healthy functioning in your cells, and it's important to maintain the proper balance of nutrients. Certain nutrients aren't effective unless taken with other nutrients. For instance, calcium needs its "buddies" magnesium and vitamin D huddled around for the calcium to be properly absorbed. If you are currently an "à la carte-r," choose a balanced vitamin and mineral supplement instead.

Supplements Aren't Regulated

One dilemma that makes it difficult to choose any sort of supplement is the fact that nutritional supplements are not regulated or routinely tested by our government. The FDA (Food and Drug Administration) does not have any control over nutritional supplements unless a blatant problem surfaces—such as serious adverse reactions. Only then do both the FDA and the Federal Trade Commission get involved, which leave us without the normal safeguards that most of us take for granted. Instead we have many companies making extraordinary claims about various supplements, such as "lose weight overnight" or "reverse aging" or "boost your sex drive." No agency is making sure that what is in the bottle is the same as what is listed on the label of the bottle. Or that it will do what the label says it does. In studies done on various supplements to test whether the product ingredients matched the label, results showed that some products do not even contain what is listed on the label. Some have far too much of an active ingredient. And some had very little of the ingredients listed on the label. And some even had dangerous ingredients! For example, ConsumerLab tested twenty-one ginseng products. Seven contained less than the listed amount of ginseng. Nearly half contained high levels of lead or pesticides![6]

Keep this in mind and be cautious about supplements, especially those that make outlandish claims that seem too good to be true. Stick with big-name brands and specialized companies that prove they test their products.

A great online resource for various brands of nutritional supplements that have been tested and "passed their exams" is an independent testing company called ConsumerLab, at www.ConsumerLab.com. The company offers some information free of charge and, for a small fee, will allow you to read unlimited reviews.

Supplements That "Boost Energy"

Many nonvitamin/nonmineral supplements on the market claim to boost your energy and relieve fatigue, but do they? And at what cost to your health? And your bank account? If the product is safe but not effective, you've only lost the money you spent. The cost to your health is the biggest issue, because if a supplement is potentially dangerous, you may be seriously affected, or even die, from using it! Some might think that sounds overly dramatic; all we're talking about are herbs and other "natural" substances, right? But herbs and natural supplements contain active substances, and when they are consumed some can be very dangerous.

> *"What natural substance can I get to increase my energy?"*

"Energizing" Ephedra = Danger

The most dangerous natural "energy" supplement is called *ephedra* or *Ma Huang.* It is used not only for energy but also to aid in weight loss and to improve athletic performance. Many very fit athletes have literally dropped dead after workouts while being on ephedra-containing supplements, and the FDA has received reports of thousands of others having suffered high blood pressure, heart attacks, strokes, irregular heart rhythms, or severe psychiatric reactions, such as psychosis, when using ephedra supplements. This dangerous supplement is commonly found in diet aids claiming to boost your metabolism, such as Hydroxycut, Metabolife 356, and Ripped Fuel. The National Institutes of Health recently did a survey of gym-goers and found that 26 percent of those in the sample had used ephedra-containing athletic products. Applying those figures to the rest of the U.S. means there could be as many as three million people using these products on a regular basis.[7] The risk appears to be highest when ephedra is combined with caffeine or another stimulant, such as guarana or kola nut, which it often is. Sometimes ephedra or Ma Huang are hard to find on the label, so you may need look for this ingredient under "proprietary blend."

I advise you *not* to take any supplement product containing ephedra or Ma Huang. This is a potent stimulant that raises blood pressure and speeds the heartbeat, which can strain your heart and blood vessels. Although you may have the sensation of more energy briefly, it is more likely you will feel overstimulated. Another reason to avoid these products is that, since these products are not regulated, you cannot depend on the label to tell you how much ephedra is in each dose. A study at the University of Arkansas tested twenty different brands of ephedra-containing herbal dietary supplements. The study found in many products a variation of more than 20 percent between what the label said and what was actually inside the capsule. The amount of ephedra in one brand varied by 260 percent from one lot to the next. And one brand did not contain any ephedra![8]

Safer Stimulants

Several other natural stimulants are, for the most part, not a health concern, but as with any stimulant, they are likely to increase your heart rate and may increase your blood pressure. The "energy" that these stimulants give you is artificial; you are not energized because you have improved your nutritional status, but because your brain and body are being directly stimulated. These stimulants include *guarana* (commonly found in soft drinks and teas in Brazil and now in certain supplement drinks and diet aids in the U.S.), *kola nut,* and *caffeine* as found in natural green tea, black tea, and coffee. Be on the lookout for these natural stimulants in the many supplement "energy" drinks made by companies such as Sobe and Snapple.

Ginseng is also commonly added to such drinks (also available as a supplement bought as tea, in capsule form, and as dried root) because it too is said to increase energy, improve your mood, strengthen the immune system, and even spice up your sex life. The claims for energy and invigoration have been confirmed by some studies, but the studies on ginseng have not confirmed all the other claims. Also, be aware that ginseng may not be safe for pregnant or nursing women, children, and those on certain medications like steroids and antidepressants.[9]

What Supplements Were in My Cereal This Morning?

In addition to vitamins and minerals, be on the lookout when reading your food label for a whole host of other supplements, such as *ginkgo biloba, Saint John's wort, carnitine, echinacea,* and *dong quai*—all with claims that vary from helping to prevent colds to fighting depression to relieving menopausal symptoms.[10] These show up especially in those "natural supplement" drinks, but also are in cereals, nutrition bars, even corn chips, and other foods.

Don't Overdo It

Nearly half of adults take nutritional supplements, and now many foods and drinks are fortified with supplements. If you are taking both, there is a real possibility that you may be accidentally overdosing on certain supplements. The saying that you can't have too much of a good thing does not apply to nutritional supplements. Too much of certain supplements could prove toxic to your body. For example, if you take a calcium supplement, and drink calcium-fortified orange juice, and eat Total cereal with calcium—you may have swallowed your upper intake limit for calcium at breakfast alone.

Toothbrush Reminder

With vitamin and mineral supplements, it is not only important to consider *what* you take, and *how much* you take, but also *how* and *when* you take them. It is best to take your vitamins and minerals with food to minimize stomach upset and maximize your absorption of nutrients, especially the fat-soluble vitamins A, D, E, and K. But the supplement cannot help you if you don't remember to take it. I recommend you put your supplement right by your toothbrush, and when you brush your teeth after breakfast, take your supplements. If yours is a twice-a-day formulation, take the other dose after dinner or at bedtime, whenever you brush your teeth.

Don't Hide the Bottles under a Bushel

Please don't hide your use of supplements from your doctor or other health care provider. Even if you think your doctor may not support your choice to use supplements, provide your doctor with a list of what is in each one, or simply bring in the bottles of each supplement. Nutritional supplements interact with many medications, sometimes increasing the effect of the medicines, other times decreasing their effect, so your doctor needs to know.

This is *crucial* when you are going to have surgery. Most herbs could cause complications either during or after surgery. Because of this major concern, the American Medical Association has issued the following guidelines outlining possible complications and which herbs need to be stopped up to a week prior to surgery:[11]

- Bleeding: garlic (1 week), ginseng (1 week), ginkgo biloba (1 1/2 days)
- Heart and blood pressure instability: ephedra (1 week)
- Too much sedation: kava kava (1 day), valerian (5–7 days)
- Drug interactions and bleeding: St. John's wort (5 days)
- Immunity suppression (if taken for 8 weeks or more): echinacea (5–7 days)

WARNING: *Always* tell your doctor and anesthesiologist what herbs and supplements you are taking, because they may want you to stop them even earlier.

Glucosamine—Potentially Energetic for Your Joints

Glucosamine may not boost your energy level directly, but studies confirm that it reduces joint pain, increases joint function, and decreases the loss of cartilage in those with osteoarthritis.[12] For many, it is as effective as anti-inflammatory drugs like ibuprofen.[13] So, after taking 1,500 mg per day, for anywhere from a week to many weeks, you may find your pain and stiffness have decreased and that you can do more physical activities. To continue the benefits if you find it effective, you must continue the glucosamine. The recommended types to take are glucosamine hydrochloride (most potent form) and glucosamine sulfate.

Help for Adverse Supplement Reactions

If you have a problem or bad side effect as a result of taking a nutritional supplement, report it to the FDA by sending in a Med Watch report. The only way the FDA can control a dietary supplement is if the product is proven harmful, so the FDA needs to know if you have experienced any harmful or unusual effects. You can obtain a form to mail or fax by calling Med Watch (1-800-332-1088). Or submit it online at the Med Watch website, www.fda.gov/medwatch.

The Federal Trade Commission (FTC) also watches for fraud and harmful products and accepts reports of adverse reactions. Call the FTC at (877) FTC-HELP, or go to the FTC website, www.ftc.gov.

Energy in a Bottle?

Are you looking to find reliable energy in a bottle? Now you know the closest thing we have that can truly boost your energy is a daily multivitamin-mineral supplement. Even the American Medical Association is recommending them now! Remember, supplements cannot replace the nutrition we get from food, but they can improve our nutritional state—and our energy levels—when we take them regularly and eat healthy.

5

Weight-Loss Strategies That Are Wise and Energize

Have you been trying to lose weight but aren't happy with your progress? You're not alone. Weight loss was the second highest ranked issue of concern and the second highest ranked topic moms asked questions about in the MOPS Moms Health Survey. Weight is also a major issue for our country as a whole. In the year 2000, nearly one in every five adults in the U.S. fits the criteria for being "obese." This is a 61 percent increase in the rate of obesity in just nine years! The same study found that nearly 60 percent of Americans fit the criteria for being overweight.[1] But the 2002 Harris Poll found that 33 percent of U.S. adults over twenty-five are obese, and 80 percent are overweight![2] If you are ready to lose your excess weight, join me now in our MOPS Spa Strategy Room, where together we will tackle the issue of which weight-loss plan will work best for you.

"What is the best way to lose and maintain a healthy weight?"

The Basics of a Wise Weight-Loss Plan

To lose weight you need to change at least one thing in your everyday life. I know that sounds basic and almost too simple, but how many of us like to imagine that one day we will wake up to find that, without making any lifestyle changes, our extra weight has just slipped off our hips and is nowhere to be found. This old adage is true: "If you keep doing what you've been doing, you'll keep getting what you've been getting."

We need to take action. But what action should that be? And what plan? It is very important that the program be a healthy and wise weight-loss plan. But the most important key to weight-loss success is finding the plan that works for *you*. If you will not or cannot stick with a weight-loss plan, you will be discouraged and stop trying.

What Is Your Target Healthy Weight?

First, you need to figure out your target healthy weight. The best way to do this is to calculate your BMI (Body Mass Index), which is determined from your height and current weight. Once you have those measurements, you can either do the calculation yourself, find it using the Body Mass Index Table (next page), or log on to the National Institutes of Health website at www.nhlbisupport.com/bmi, where the calculation will be done for you. Get your *real* weight and height measurements and let's get started!

Here's how you calculate your BMI (you need your current weight in pounds and your height in inches):

1. Take your weight in pounds
2. Divide it by your height in inches
3. Then divide that number again by your height in inches
4. Then multiply that number by 703

You should have a BMI number between 18 and 40. What does it mean? Here are the determinations from the National Institutes of Health:

- Underweight = <18.5
- Normal weight = 18.5–24.9

Body Mass Index Table

	Normal						Overweight					Obese										Extreme Obesity														
BMI	19	20	21	22	23	24	25	26	27	28	29	30	31	32	33	34	35	36	37	38	39	40	41	42	43	44	45	46	47	48	49	50	51	52	53	54
Height (inches)	Body Weight (pounds)																																			
58	91	96	100	105	110	115	119	124	129	134	138	143	148	153	158	162	167	172	177	181	186	191	196	201	205	210	215	220	224	229	234	239	244	248	253	258
59	94	99	104	109	114	119	124	128	133	138	143	148	153	158	163	168	173	178	183	188	193	198	203	208	212	217	222	227	232	237	242	247	252	257	262	267
60	97	102	107	112	118	123	128	133	138	143	148	153	158	163	168	174	179	184	189	194	199	204	209	215	220	225	230	235	240	245	250	255	261	266	271	276
61	100	106	111	116	122	127	132	137	143	148	153	158	164	169	174	180	185	190	195	201	206	211	217	222	227	232	238	243	248	254	259	264	269	275	280	285
62	104	109	115	120	126	131	136	142	147	153	158	164	169	175	180	186	191	196	202	207	213	218	224	229	235	240	246	251	256	262	267	273	278	284	289	295
63	107	113	118	124	130	135	141	146	152	158	163	169	175	180	186	191	197	203	208	214	220	225	231	237	242	248	254	259	265	270	278	282	287	293	299	304
64	110	116	122	128	134	140	145	151	157	163	169	174	180	186	192	197	204	209	215	221	227	232	238	244	250	256	262	267	273	279	285	291	296	302	308	314
65	114	120	126	132	138	144	150	156	162	168	174	180	186	192	198	204	210	216	222	228	234	240	246	252	258	264	270	276	282	288	294	300	306	312	318	324
66	118	124	130	136	142	148	155	161	167	173	179	186	192	198	204	210	216	223	229	235	241	247	253	260	266	272	278	284	291	297	303	309	315	322	328	334
67	121	127	134	140	146	153	159	166	172	178	185	191	198	204	211	217	223	230	236	242	249	255	261	268	274	280	287	293	299	306	312	319	325	331	338	344
68	125	131	138	144	151	158	164	171	177	184	190	197	203	210	216	223	230	236	243	249	256	262	269	276	282	289	295	302	308	315	322	328	335	341	348	354
69	128	135	142	149	155	162	169	176	182	189	196	203	209	216	223	230	236	243	250	257	263	270	277	284	291	297	304	311	318	324	331	338	345	351	358	365
70	132	139	146	153	160	167	174	181	188	195	202	209	216	222	229	236	243	250	257	264	271	278	285	292	299	306	313	320	327	334	341	348	355	362	369	376
71	136	143	150	157	165	172	179	186	193	200	208	215	222	229	236	243	250	257	265	272	279	286	293	301	308	315	322	329	338	343	351	358	365	372	379	386
72	140	147	154	162	169	177	184	191	199	206	213	221	228	235	242	250	258	265	272	279	287	294	302	309	316	324	331	338	346	353	361	368	375	383	390	397
73	144	151	159	166	174	182	189	197	204	212	219	227	235	242	250	257	265	272	280	288	295	302	310	318	325	333	340	348	355	363	371	378	386	393	401	408
74	148	155	163	171	179	186	194	202	210	218	225	233	241	249	256	264	272	280	287	295	303	311	319	326	334	342	350	358	365	373	381	389	396	404	412	420
75	152	160	168	176	184	192	200	208	216	224	232	240	248	256	264	272	279	287	295	303	311	319	327	335	343	351	359	367	375	383	391	399	407	415	423	431
76	156	164	172	180	189	197	205	213	221	230	238	246	254	263	271	279	287	295	304	312	320	328	336	344	353	361	369	377	385	394	402	410	418	426	435	443

- Overweight = 25–29.9
- Obesity = 30 or greater

A BMI between 18 and 25 has been considered healthy, but new data found the most benefits in the lower range. According to the National Heart, Lung, and Blood Institute Obesity Education Initiative, "New data shows that your health risks decrease if you're at the lower end of the BMI spectrum—from about 18 to 22."[3]

So what is right for you? Depending on your bone structure, your ideal weight may be at the lower or higher end of the 18 to 25 range. Your wrist measurement will give you your best clue whether you have a larger, smaller, or average-sized body frame. If your wrist is less than 6 inches, you are likely "small boned," or if over 6.25 inches you are likely "large boned." Smaller-boned women probably are healthier at the lower end of the healthy weight BMI range (18–22), while larger-boned women may find the top of the range more realistic (22–25). If you are very muscular, your right weight is likely at the high end of the range. As we age we usually drift toward the higher end of the range too.

Now measure your waist. If your waist measurement is 35 inches or greater (35 inches for women, 40 inches for men), and you are *not* pregnant or recently postpartum, your health may be in danger. As we discussed in chapter 2, such a measurement usually indicates a lot of internal, or intra-abdominal, fat, which is linked with serious health issues or the metabolic syndrome. It is also a strong clue that you are secreting a lot of cortisol, probably from excessive and chronic emotional stress. It's a warning that you need to see your doctor for an evaluation.

What are the health risks for those whose weight is "out of range" or who have significant intra-abdominal fat stores? It depends on whether you have other risk factors:[4]

- High blood pressure (hypertension)
- High LDL cholesterol ("bad" cholesterol)
- Low HDL cholesterol ("good" cholesterol)
- High triglycerides
- High blood glucose (sugar)

- Family history of premature heart disease
- Physical inactivity
- Cigarette smoking

If you have two or more of these risk factors, and a BMI of 25–29 (overweight) or higher, or if you have a waist measurement of 35 inches or greater (women) when not pregnant, it is strongly recommended that you lose weight. Research shows that you have an increased risk of developing high blood pressure, high blood cholesterol, type 2 diabetes, heart disease, stroke, and certain cancers. As you look over these lists, if you find your health may now be in significant danger, the good news is that even a mild to moderate amount of weight loss can significantly decrease your risk. So every pound lost counts as health gained!

With this in mind, look at the BMI table again and see whether you agree with the ideal weight range that corresponds with your body type and measurements. Does it seem right to you? Then pick the weight in that range that you know to be a reasonable goal. Just remember that you won't reach your goal overnight, but you may sooner than you think.

Look at What You've Been Eating

The next step is to be honest about what you've been eating. This is the place to start if you want to improve your diet and lose weight. Are you eating regular meals? Skipping meals? Are you eating a healthy balance of foods as was discussed in chapter 3? What time of day are you loading up on calories? All these questions will be easy to answer after you track your eating for a week. Take a notepad and write down everything you eat for that week. Don't forget to include those pre-dinner samplings while you're cooking, the few mouthfuls of leftover pudding, and the late-night snacks. Also get an idea of the quantities of foods you eat. And note whether you're hungry or just eating on automatic. This diary is for *your* benefit, so you don't have to show it to anyone. Be as honest as possible so you get the most benefit from this exercise.

Identify Your "Can't Live without It" Foods

As you look over your food diary, do certain foods leap out at you as foods you can't imagine eliminating from your diet? Foods like chocolate, ice cream, cookies, chips, and pizza? These are often the very foods we feel must go if we are to lose weight—because many diets say so. But I am a firm believer that if your weight-loss plan eliminates too many of your favorite foods, you will not stick with it. In fact, you may actually eat larger quantities of these foods because they are now "forbidden." No food is forbidden in this approach, but you need to be reasonable about the quantity you eat.

The recent success of the "Ice Cream Diet" is a great example of how *not* eliminating your favorite food can help you succeed at losing weight. The folks at *Prevention* magazine developed this diet. It allows you to add to their basic plan up to 1 cup of ice cream per day. When you look at the basic plan, it is a wise, balanced, and healthy eating plan that counts the ice cream as one of the diet's sources of calcium but, more importantly, adds ice cream as the treat that keeps you with the plan.

So what should your diet plan be called? "The Piece-of-Chocolate-a-Day Diet" or "The Pizza-Once-a-Week Diet"? Figure out what food or foods still need to be in your diet (in sensible amounts) so that you will not feel deprived.

Spending Those Calories

The basic requirement for weight loss is that you must take in fewer calories than you burn in a day. For most women, the rule of thumb is to decrease your calorie intake by 500 calories a day to lose a sensible one to two pounds per week. That leaves most of you with 1,500 to 1,800 calories a day that you can spend. How will you spend your calories? And where will you shave off the 500 calories each day? Here are some pointers to spending wisely and finding a healthy diet that provides plenty of energy:

Spread your calories out over the entire day. You won't be as hungry.

There shall be no skipping of meals. Did you know you can eat more and end up losing weight? But if you forget to eat and end up skipping more than the occasional meal (whether by accident or on purpose), you may be sabotaging your metabolism. Your body will think you are starving, causing your metabolism to slow down to conserve energy. It will now be harder to lose weight because you are burning fewer calories! Instead of skipping meals, you should eat at least three meals a day, which revs up your metabolism, and the pounds come off much more easily. Of course, it also matters *what* you eat during those meals.

Eat breakfast. Eating breakfast is one of the four most common behaviors of 3,000 "successful losers" who have kept the weight off after losing an average of 66 pounds each.[5] Breakfast eaters jump-start their metabolism so they burn more calories throughout the day and have better concentration. But studies show that more than 33 percent of individuals skip breakfast at least once a week, while more than 20 percent skip breakfast five or more times a week.[6] Please don't skip breakfast!

Snacks are very important. They keep you from feeling hungry and overeating at meals. Just make sure each snack is a healthy snack.

Don't eliminate all fats or all carbohydrates. As we discussed in chapter 3, diet plans that tell you to eliminate a food group are *not* wise. You need a reasonable amount of fat (mono- and polyunsaturated) in your diet for good health, and fat takes longer to go through your system, so you feel full longer. Carbohydrates are your greatest source of fuel, but lean toward the whole grains and complex carbohydrates more than sugars and simple carbohydrates.

Try to eat "heavier" foods earlier in the day. If you "eat breakfast like a king, lunch like a prince, and dinner like a pauper," you will have the chance to burn off those extra calories earlier in the day.[7]

Don't forget to include your favorite food. If done within reason, this helps you stay with your weight-loss plan.

Smart Ways to Shave Off 500 Calories a Day

Consider portion sizes. Some moms can achieve this cutback merely by decreasing the portion sizes of their usual foods.

Consider using a healthy meal-replacement drink or bar for one meal a day. Studies show this to be an effective way for many folks to make the calorie cut and stay with it for the long haul. The use of a nutrient-fortified, liquid meal-replacement drink in place of one or two meals per day was reviewed in two recent studies, and both showed the groups that used the drinks lost more weight than the groups who followed 1,200 to 1,500 calorie diets with instruction from dieticians or doctors.[8] One of those studies also found that using a meal-replacement drink once a day helped participants maintain their weight loss over a four-year period.[9] This is a good choice only if you are diligent about getting your other nutrients at the other meals, such as getting at least five servings a day of fruits and vegetables, plus healthy amounts of protein, fat, and carbohydrates.

Slim-Fast is the most common meal replacement on the market, but when you look over the fine print of its food label you may find the contents are not the healthy mix we desire. A healthy meal-replacement drink would have fructose for a carbohydrate source (instead of only sugar or corn syrup), and soy or whey for protein sources. Drinks that fit these standards and taste great include Revival's soy drink, Kashi's Go LEAN, Melaleuca's Attain, USANA's Nutrimeal, and Quixtar's Trim Advantage, to name a few.

Eat "boring" food. Cutting back on food intake often is easier if the foods you eat are limited in variety and, well, boring. Beware the curse of the all-you-can-eat buffet where you have dozens of food choices. You will almost definitely eat more there than if you had a less exciting choice of foods.

Exercise. This choice is a triple bonus for anyone on a weight-loss plan. You burn calories. You build muscle (and every added pound of muscle burns an extra thirty-five to fifty calories a day). In addition, exercise directly increases your metabolism. If you are exercising regularly, you may not have to shave off as many calories from your diet to still lose weight.

What Do You Need to Keep You on Track?

When choosing a weight-loss plan, one of the most important factors to keep in mind is whether the plan will provide the support you need to help you stick with it. Here are some common factors that can help you stay on a weight-loss program:

Accountability. There is usually more success when you have to keep track of all you eat, weigh in front of others each week, or even just talk with someone who is keeping you accountable. Information pooled from twenty-nine different weight-loss studies shows that those participants who were given very specific instructions on meal-planning and were held accountable during the plan kept off an average of seven pounds when weighed five years later.[10]

Prepackaged foods. Many successful weight-loss plans, such as Nutri-System, Jenny Craig, and to some degree Weight Watchers, utilize prepackaged meals to control portion size, offer a nutritionally balanced low-calorie meal, and help you stick with it because it's easy to figure out what you should eat. Research confirms that this is a highly effective approach for many women. In fact, a recent study found that those who ate the meals provided as part of the plan lost more weight than those who did not use the food provided.[11]

Emotional and spiritual support. Sticking with a weight-loss plan can be challenging, so make sure there is enough support in your corner cheering you on and picking you up when you are down.

Realistic goals. A wise and healthy approach to weight loss is one that strives for a weight loss of one to two pounds per week. Those that promise shedding ten to twenty pounds in a weekend are to be avoided. Set little goals. Remind yourself that your health will benefit from even tiny increments of weight loss.

Permission to "blow-it" a few times. Because you went off your diet plan an occasional time does not mean you "failed." Just let it go and get back on the plan.

Worthy Weight-Loss Plans

It is time to choose your plan. You know your target weight. You know you need to cut 500 calories per day. You know you can't live without food. And you now have a better sense of what factors will keep you on track. There's one more thing. I recommend checking with your doctor before beginning any weight-loss program, particularly if you have any known health issues.

With the knowledge you have, you could "do it yourself" without any formal program, but for most women, doing this with a friend to keep each other accountable is more effective.

> *"What diet methods are safe? Are low-carbohydrate diets healthy?"*

Here are a few of the programs I recommend (there are undoubtedly other worthy programs that I could recommend that are not listed here, so if you know of one that you want to consider, use the principles in this chapter to find out if it fits our criteria):

First Place. This is a Christian weight-loss plan that combines spiritual growth with weight loss. They hold weekly meetings, usually at a local church, and use a very sound diet and exercise plan along with high accountability and support. Contact www.firstplace.org or call 1-800-727-5223 to locate a group in your area or to begin your own church group.

New Life Ministry's Lose it for Life plan, Thin Within, 3D Christian Diet, and Weigh Down Workshop. These are other Christian-based weight-loss plans worth considering.[12]

Weight Watchers. With weekly meetings that include weigh-in accountability and support, education, an easy-to-follow diet plan, and low-cost membership fee. A two-year-long research study found that those studied in the WW group (as compared to a group using a do-it-yourself weight-loss plan) lost more weight and kept off 78 percent of the pounds lost when weighed two years later.[13] Contact WW through their universal phone number (1-800-651-6000) or go to their website (www.weightwatchers.com) and enroll as a member. You then commit to going weekly to a Weight Watchers weigh-in/support meeting in your area. For those who cannot attend weekly meetings, Weight Watchers offers an on-line membership option.

Jenny Craig. This organization offers emotional support and personalized counseling, prepackaged meals, and charges fees for services. Eventually you will learn to get the same results eating "normal" food. Contact one of the 652 Weight Loss Centres worldwide, or you can join via the Internet at www.jennycraig.com.

Nutri-System. Uses prepackaged foods supplemented by your own fresh dairy products and veggies. Online support counselors are available, but there is no in-person accountability. Contact www.nutrisystem.com for more information.

"Aim for a Healthy Weight" plan. This can be found on National Institutes of Health website. An excellent resource that offers sample reduced-calorie menus, tips on exercise, and calculates your BMI. Go to www.nhlbi.nih.gov/health/public/heart/obesity/lose_wt/index.htm.

DASH diet (Dietary Approaches to Stop Hypertension). This do-it-yourself diet plan was developed to provide a healthy diet to help people decrease their blood pressure, but is a sound eating plan for anyone. It is especially good for weight loss since it is low in saturated fat, cholesterol, and total fat, and high in fruits, vegetables, and whole grains. Salt intake is reduced to between 1.5 and 2.5 grams per day. You can get a free copy of the diet and sample menus online at www.nhlbi.nih.gov/health/public/heart/hbp/dash/new_dash.pdf.[14]

The "Ice Cream Diet." This is a very sound diet plan that closely resembles the healthy DASH diet. It is outlined in detail in the book *The Ice Cream Diet* by Holly McCord, the nutrition editor of *Prevention* magazine. Also available: *The Peanut Butter Diet,* with a similar approach by Holly McCord.

Diet Danger Zone

When "weight panic" hits, it is tempting to quickly try the fad that promises the fastest weight loss with the least amount of effort, or to just drastically cut calorie intake, or even quit eating meals all together. But there is a reason why such choices are called "crash diets." These plans usually are quick to fail, which makes you even more discouraged and may even send you to finish off the leftover birthday cake. Don't "crash and burn" by resorting to such methods. Here are several diets you should avoid:

The Atkins Diet, Sugar Busters, Carbohydrate Addict's Diet, Somersize, Protein Power. The confusing thing about these diets is that you probably will lose weight on these plans (at least initially), because these diets all severely limit carbohydrates, which makes you lose a lot of water at first. But of even more concern is the high concentration of saturated fat in these diets, which make them very heart-*un*healthy! These high-protein, high-fat diet programs do not limit the amount of animal protein and animal fat you consume. These diets severely limit the kinds of foods allowed, though there are no limits on quantities. In the early phases of several of these plans no fruit is allowed and meals have low fiber intake and few veggies. Because of this unhealthy balance of foods there is a potential risk of increased coronary artery disease, gout, kidney stones, increased kidney disease, and inadequate intake of nutrients. Some or all of these plans have been condemned by a variety of respected health groups, including the American Heart Association, American Dietetic Association, the United States Department of Agriculture, American College of Sports Medicine, Women's Sports Foundation, the Cooper Sports Foundation, and the Center for Science in the Public Interest.[15]

The Blood-Type Diet. The truth is, there is no scientific basis for this diet and no studies to confirm that anything it proposes is true. This diet eliminates many healthful foods from your diet. But the banned foods are solely selected by your blood type. This is as absurd as saying, "all blue-eyed people must not eat corn!" there are no research findings that support any of these food bans or blood-type diet claims.

Diet Aids: Should I—or Shouldn't I?

Whether you go into a drugstore, a regular grocery store, or a health food store, once you find the right aisle you will find shelves packed with assorted diet aids. All claim to make weight loss easy, and a large proportion claim they are an all "natural" weight-loss solution. But many diet aids are dangerous to use, including "all natural" ones, and do more harm than good. You need to know more before taking one of those diet-aid bottles to the checkout register.

If you wish to try a diet aid, you need to know how that particular aid will act on your body before you try it. Most diet aids fall into at least one of these four categories:

1. Speed up your metabolism
2. Suppress your appetite
3. Block absorption of food or calories
4. Do nothing

Stimulants

Stimulants are the most dangerous diet aids. Although most stimulants do not cause serious harm, with some the side effect can be death with the first dose!

Ephedra (or Ma Huang). Often billed as a "natural weight-loss aid," its action is more amphetamine-like and dangerous. As discussed in chapter 4, ephedra use is associated with many deaths, heart attacks, strokes, and psychosis in previously healthy people. Does that mean everyone will have difficulty with it? No. Research confirms that some people report great results without side effects.[16] But there is currently no way to tell which ephedra users will have a fatal reaction and which will live to fit into a smaller dress size. Since you may be risking your life with this diet aid, don't use it.

Guarana (Paullinia cupana). A natural stimulant and appetite suppressant with the "reputation for lifting mood without the edginess of coffee." It is also said to provide "a longer period of stimulation because it moves more slowly through the digestive system than coffee."[17]

Caffeine. Used in dieting to suppress appetite and speed metabolism.

Apple Cider Vinegar Capsules. The theory behind this ineffective diet aid is that vinegar will "boost your metabolism and help your body get rid of stored fat." But there is no scientific evidence to back these claims.[18]

Appetite Suppressants

Citrimax (fruit from Garcinia cambogia). Citrimax appears to suppress appetite for some users; it appears to be safe. It also claims to inhibit fat production with the active ingredient hydroxycitric acid, but evidence is weak on that claim, with no effect found in a well-done clinical study.[19] It may, however, help you to not regain weight.[20]

CLA (Conjugated Linoleic Acid). Some users report that their appetite is less when taking this product. But the big controversy is about whether or not this supplement makes people lose fat and gain lean muscle instead, since it works that way in animal studies. So far, most of the research on humans says no.[21]

Prescription drugs such as Meridia also work by suppressing appetite.

Food Absorption Blockers

With these diet aids, supposedly more of what you eat is excreted rather than being absorbed by the body and turned into fat.

Fat Blockers, Chitosan. A natural product made from the hard covering, or chitin, of shellfish. It claims to trap the fat in food you have just eaten while the fat is still in your digestive tract, then carry it out in your stool. But effectiveness is not consistent. A well-done study in England found no weight reduction after four weeks of treatment in the group using chitosan.[22] If you use this product, a concern is that the fat-soluble vitamins you just ate could also be trapped and taken out with the "trash." This product could also give you diarrhea. Those allergic to shellfish may be allergic to this product.

> *"In all these things we are more than conquerors through him who loved us."*
>
> — *Romans 8:37*

Carbohydrate Blockers. In theory, this product made from white kidney beans or soybeans is supposed to cause the starch you just ate to not be broken down into simple sugars—so it won't be absorbed in your body. But the results do not match the claims. One study was done on female rats in which the rats were given potato (starch) for four weeks with different amounts of the "starch blocker"—including a dose that in theory should have blocked 100 percent of the starch. Yet the rats showed no weight loss at any level of the blocker. Researchers did find measurable losses of copper and zinc because of this supplement.[23]

Remember, when it comes to diet aids, new fad diet plans, and $10 "gold" watches, if it sounds too good to be true, it probably is!

Postpartum Weight-Loss Blues

If you are a new mom and need to lose some weight, I know this can be hard on your self-esteem. But let's put this in perspective. Your body has just undergone the most radical transformation that God intended for any human body, and somehow you are supposed to accept that this is no big deal. Your body mass likely changed by about 25 percent in only a few months. Then, just as dramatically, your body started changing back after you heard your baby's welcoming wail. It is utterly miraculous what God equipped moms' bodies to do in this short time, and even more miraculous that our bodies return pretty close to "normal" after all these changes.

The truth is, it is going to take some time for things to return to normal. It took a while for that weight to get there, and it is going to take a while for it to leave. This is a time when we have to wait for the weight to come off. There's an old saying, "Nine months on, nine months off."

If you are breastfeeding, you may see the first pounds slip away fairly quickly. But it is very common for those last ten pounds to not budge until you *stop* breastfeeding. Your body may be holding on to them as a protective reserve so that you have enough body fat to make milk if your food supply runs out.

Beware the extreme ends of the new-mommy-eating spectrum: from the "I am so exhausted and sleep deprived I've got to eat everything in sight" end, to the "I want to lose this weight *now* so I'll not eat anything" end. Especially if you are breastfeeding, be certain that you do not radically reduce your calorie or nutrient intake. When friends or family members call after the baby is born and say, "What can we do?" ask them to bring you a healthy meal or two, or a couple casseroles that you can freeze and bring out when you need them. It will make them feel good that they could help, and this will truly help you during this amazing time of adjustment.

Moms, be patient with your body and the process of transformation that is still happening in the months after your pregnancy. This is one miracle that takes a bit of time.

You Can Do it!

The state of your weight does not determine your worth, but it can greatly impact your physical health. If you are not currently at your best weight, I encourage you to begin a weight-loss plan most suitable for you. Now you know your ideal weight range and have read through the factors that make up a safe and effective weight-loss plan. It is time to take action.

Keep in mind that losing excess weight does not happen overnight. Remember that, especially if your weight holds steady for a few weeks. Dropping those extra pounds is one of the best things you can do for your health, your state of mind, and your outlook. Just take it a day at a time and you will succeed!

6

Exercise—A Necessary Key to the Energy You Need

Whew! Boy, did I need that! You see, I was feeling stressed out after a hectic day, and it was time to meet with you to devise your personal exercise plan. But first I had to get rid of my stress. Even though I didn't have time for a full workout, I exercised. I just turned on some "Oldie's" rock-and-roll and danced around the living room with abandon until I found joy in the music. Then I cooled down with a couple of relaxation exercises. Now, just twenty minutes from when I started, I feel so much better! In fact, I feel like a new person. It is amazing what even a few minutes of exercise can do for you!

Most Moms Are *Not* Working Out

We are so blessed to have exercise as an option. But unfortunately one of the most significant findings in the MOPS Moms Health Survey was that 76 percent of all the moms surveyed say they do *not* work out. Other surveys also confirm that lack of exercise—such as the recent nationwide survey that found 55 percent of adults in the U.S. do not exercise on a regular basis.[1]

The MOPS Moms Health Survey also found that 84 percent of all surveyed moms ranked their need for more energy as one of their top five issues, and 60 percent ranked losing weight in their top five, while 64 percent ranked stress in their top five issues of concern. But of those who ranked these issues in the top five, in each category only 25 to 30 percent of these moms said they work out.

The good news is that, if you too fall into this group of non-exercisers, I can nearly guarantee that you will have more energy, feel less stressed, and likely lose weight (or at least firm what you have) once we find the right exercise that works for you. I am confident that there is *some* type of exercise you can fit into your day and even enjoy doing. You can make exercise work for *you,* and you are *not* restricted by what has typically been called "working out." It doesn't matter whether you walk, run, jump rope, climb stairs, swim, row, bicycle, dance, stand on your head, go to the gym, do Pilates, use an exercise video, take the kids for a brisk stroller walk, or play tennis, baseball, basketball, or even Ping-Pong—as long as you get up and move! If you think you hate to exercise, look over this list and see if there's anything you haven't yet tried. Or maybe you'll see something you used to enjoy. If an activity looks interesting, give it a try! The most important thing to do is to start. Even if you can exercise for only five minutes, I'm asking you to do just that. Trust me. It will be worth it to begin. Let's look at some of the reasons why exercise is well worth the effort.

Why Exercise?

If I had to give you just one reason to exercise, it would be to prevent the harm that stress can cause. "Exercise is the ultimate neutralizer of the effects of stress," says Dr. Pamela Peeke, a former researcher at the National Institutes of Health and author of the book *Fight Fat after Forty.* "During vigorous exercise, the body secretes biochemicals called *beta endorphins,* which calm you down and decrease the levels of stress hormones in your body."[2] With lower levels of stress hormones coursing through your system (cortisol in particular), you are less likely to gain the dangerous intra-abdominal fat and less likely to get the metabolic syndrome we discussed in chapter 2. You'll recall that when high levels of stress hormones are continually released into your body, cortisol makes you store fat specifically inside your abdomen. This can lead to heart disease, high blood pressure, and diabetes.

Exercise gives you abundant, immediate gratification: it burns calories, relieves stress, decreases anxiety, boosts both your mood and energy level, and improves sexual function (especially arousal). But it also brings benefits that are less obvious—for example, it increases the good HDL cholesterol and improves immune response—and these affect how long you might be around to enjoy your life.[3] The long-term benefits of exercise include:

- Builds muscle. This makes you stronger and leaner.
- Increases your metabolism 24/7. For every pound of muscle you add to your body, you burn 35 to 50 more calories each day.
- Helps fight obesity. Exercising builds muscle while burning fat.
- Strengthens cardiovascular system, especially your heart.
- Decreases bone loss and osteoporosis (severe bone loss).
- Strengthens your immune system.
- Improves your overall function (particularly in those with fibromyalgia, arthritis, and diabetes).
- Helps prevent diseases like heart disease, hypertension, and diabetes.

Some of the biggest and most recent health news was the discovery that moderate exercise helps prevent diabetes. In fact, the news was so big that the researchers stopped the study early so they could report these findings. This research study looked at patients with "pre-diabetes." Those patients who moderately exercised on a regular basis, ate a healthier diet (less saturated fat, increased fiber, and a reduced caloric intake), and lost a little weight developed full-blown type 2 diabetes less than half as often as those who did not do these healthy things on a regular basis. In this study, the exercise goal was thirty minutes a day—with a combination of weight training and aerobic/cardiovascular exercise.

All that blood circulating through our bodies during exercise does amazing things. In fact, studies show that the immune system is helped so much by exercise that "exercisers take 40–50 percent fewer sick days" from work than those who do not exercise.[4] This is especially important news for those moms who seem to catch every cold and flu virus that comes by.

When Working In the "Workout" Is *Not* Working

A lot of moms find that after they have a baby (and especially their first baby), it is very hard to get back into an exercise routine. You are overwhelmed, sleep deprived, and, on top of that, you just delivered a baby. Not only are you restricted from exercising, but your body is not too likely to be very interested in exercise for a while. In addition, it is a struggle to figure out how to "work in" working out when you have this baby (and later, a young child or children) to care for while you exercise.

Before I had my son, I regularly went to our local gym for aerobics classes. But after he arrived, I never seemed to get there. I tried using the gym childcare once, but when I returned I found the caregiver trying to give my breastfed son someone else's bottle of formula! Then I discovered some new exercise videos at our local video rental store. And from then on that became my main form of exercise. It was convenient—I could turn one on while my son napped or after he went to sleep at night. I never had to travel to tone up. And now there are exercise videos for practically every type of nonsport-related indoor fitness activity. You probably can find just the right ones for you!

Maybe some of you who say you don't work out anymore don't realize that some of your current daily activities *are* technically exercise. Or maybe you think that unless you exercise for thirty minutes straight, it doesn't count. Research shows that even exercise done in ten-minute increments is effective, and you can do several short periods of exercise in

The best resource for exercise videos is Collage Video, a company that stocks seemingly every type of exercise video or DVD. It offers "379 Air-Conditioned Workouts" to choose from. Each is described in detail on the website and in the catalog. Visit the store online at www.collagevideo.com, or call 1-800-433-6769 for a catalog or information.

a day and get full credit for your efforts. For instance, take a ten-minute walk in the morning, then later when you go to the store, park at the far end of the parking lot so you have a bit of a trek to get to the store and back. After dinner take another ten-minute walk. Those three mini-walks add up to your daily thirty minutes of exercise. You can even incorporate your children into your exercise routine, for some of those walks could be brisk kids-in-the-stroller strolls. In fact the book *Strollercize: The Workout for New Mothers* outlines a very doable and effective program for toning up after pregnancy while taking your little ones for a ride.[5]

When Your Exercise Needs to Change

The best exercise for you may change many times through your motherhood. So don't be afraid to consider other choices on the exercise smorgasbord when you become bored or if your physical needs or restrictions change. For instance, after I became ill with Ménière's disease, I could no longer walk any distance, and rigorous exercise made everything worse. Then I found Pilates exercises that I could do on my bed. Now that I am stronger, I can also dance in the living room if I hold onto a chair or cane.

The irony about trying to exercise when you have physical limitations is that this is often the time when you need the stress-relieving and energy-boosting benefits of exercise the most. So if you become physically restricted or disabled at some point, don't give up. Be willing to be creative until you find an appropriate exercise that you *can* do. A good resource is a physical therapist or occupational therapist. Ask your doctor for a visit to one of these professionals so they can design a personalized program of exercises within your physical ability.

The American Council on Exercise (ACE) polled more than 3,000 fitness professionals on what they thought were the most common mistakes people make in the gym. These items made up the Top 10 list:[6]

1. Not warming up prior to the activity
2. Not stretching enough
3. Not cooling down after any type of workout
4. Exercising too intensely
5. Not exercising intensely enough
6. Not drinking enough water
7. Consuming energy bars and sports drinks during moderate workouts
8. Lifting too much weight
9. Jerking while lifting weights
10. Leaning heavily on a stair stepper machine—rather than standing upright with good posture

The Ideal Way to Exercise

To reap the best benefits from exercise, the U.S. surgeon general recommends that you burn at least 1,000 calories per week in exercise, which translates to the following:

- Walking: 30 minutes a day, or 60 minutes 3 times a week
- Jogging: 30 minutes 3 times a week
- Swimming: 30 minutes a day, or 60 minutes 3 times a week
- Cycling: 30 minutes a day, or 60 minutes 3 times a week

One question often asked is, What type of exercise is most important? Training with weights? Aerobic/cardiovascular exercise? Or others? The answer is, All of the above.

For the ideal workout plan, I recommend you exercise thirty to sixty minutes per day. Alternate aerobic exercise every other day with strength or weight training. On the aerobic days, do brisk walking, running, swimming, bicycling, aerobics classes, or tennis. On the other days do strength- or weight-training exercises.

Aerobic exercise will help you gain a healthy heart and stamina, while strength or weight training will give you upper body strength, better posture and back support, and strong abdominal muscles and legs. Weight training also helps prevent bone loss and increases your rate of metabolism so you burn more calories day and night—even when you're sleeping.

"What is the best approach to getting back in shape?"

Strength train three days a week, always with a day of rest between workouts since the muscles actually get stronger during the recovery period, not the workout period. Strength-training exercise makes the support muscles of your body frame strong through the lifting of small hand weights, using weight or resistance machines or items like resistance bands, or even your own body weight as the resistance. Here is some important weight-lifting advice from fitness expert Kevin Makely:

> Any time you lift weights, always do so with proper posture and slow, controlled movements. Jerking the weights is a sign of improper posture and too heavy a weight choice. Practice proper posture and the rest will fall into place. It is not about the number of pounds you lift, but how you lift it.[7]

End each workout with a period of stretching exercises to protect you from injury due to tight muscles, and to protect your tight muscles from injury. Notice that I said *end* your workout with stretching exercises. Always warm up first by walking or another light activity. Never stretch cold muscles. Flexibility, or stretching, exercises not only protect the body from many avoidable injuries but they also make your body move more easily. And generally they make you feel good.

There are right ways and wrong ways to stretch. The most common stretching mistake I see is bouncing. That defeats the purpose. Instead, when you stretch, stretch a part of your body slowly and steadily until the muscles just start to be uncomfortable. Then hold it there while taking a deep breath and telling your body to "relax." Try to inch forward a bit more into the stretch, but stop if it is uncomfortable. It should not hurt. If you do this on a regular basis, even the least limber person will see progress. Fitness expert Kevin Makely advises, "My top tip for stretching: Make sure you hold the stretch for at least 30 seconds."[8] An outstanding book that outlines specific stretching exercises is *Stretching* by Bob Anderson.

The order that you do exercises also may make a difference. For instance, if your goal is to shape and define your muscles, then it's best to do your weights or toning exercises first. But if your preference is to build up your aerobic endurance, then do the aerobics first.

Always remember to drink water before, during, and after exercising, and don't let your thirst be your guide. Sports drinks, such as Gatorade, are not necessary unless you are exercising very strenuously. However, if you won't drink water but will drink a sports drink, then go get Gatorade.

Helpful Relaxation Exercises for Every Mom

As we discussed in chapter 2, relaxation exercises can rescue you when you feel very stressed, anxious, and exhausted. And if you do them regularly (preferably daily, or at least three times a week), you will decrease the amount of stress and anxiety you experience. If you're not doing the breathing exercises from chapter 2, make it a habit, starting now, to do the 4-by-4-by-4 Breather and the Tense-Release Sequence Exercise. You might also want to try this body position with deep, slow breathing. It's called the *position of ultimate rest.* You need to lie down on your back on a flat surface, with your knees bent and feet flat on the floor. Then spread your feet apart just far enough so that your knees can each lean inward until the inner sides of your knees settle comfortably against each other. You can either place your arms at your sides or relax them across your chest (as if you were giving yourself a hug). Are you comfortable? Close your eyes and breathe slowly. This is a great relaxation exercise to do after you exercise—or any time you need it.

Yoga

The issue of yoga has many Christians tied up in knots. So let's talk about it. Many Christians are opposed to the practice of yoga because the physical movements have traditionally been taught in conjunction with spiritual and meditative disciplines—all practices of the Hindu and Buddhist religions—which are not compatible with Christian beliefs.

In recent years, because some report stress relief, relaxation, and other physical benefits when they do yoga exercises, just the physical movements have been taught widely by countless instructors in classes and on videotapes. But these classes and videos are still objectionable to the majority of Christians because of the potential spiritual conflict.

What about the claims of physical benefits with yoga? Although numerous studies have suggested that regular practice of yoga exercise is associated with reduced stress and anxiety,[9] improved physical strength and flexibility, and may control medical conditions such as hypertension (high blood pressure),[10] arthritis,[11] epilepsy,[12] asthma, and chronic pain,[13] there are few controlled, randomized, well-done studies to verify these benefits.

Is there a way to get the physical benefits that some associate with yoga (such as relaxation, improved physical strength, and flexibility) without the spiritual concerns that come with yoga? Yes, I believe the Pilates exercise program is the answer and offers the same physical benefits without the spiritual conflicts. Let's look at the Pilates program now.

Pilates—Relax and Exercise at the Same Time

If I could recommend only one type of exercise to you, it would be Pilates (pronounced pih-LAH-tays). Many in the fitness world agree that the Pilates method of exercise may be the perfect exercise program. Pilates, developed by fitness expert Joseph H. Pilates in the early 1900s, combines stretching and strengthening exercises. What sets it apart is the fact that you accomplish all three components of exercise within a Pilates workout, yet overall, during the series of exercises, you feel relaxed and not heavily taxed. That is a bonus for every mom! It's an efficient program that does not require a large amount of time, another bonus for moms. Plus it is perfect for women at any level of fitness. But one of the best reasons to do Pilates is that its main purpose is to strengthen your body's core support muscles. You end up with a balanced, stronger body with good posture, which protects you from all sorts of potential injuries, the kind of protection every mom can use.

There are several ways to do Pilates. You can do the exercises on a floor mat at home with an instruction book or video as a guide, attend a class that uses floor-mat exercises, or use a large resistance machine at a gym or at home. The machine is now available in home versions, two of which are called the Pilates Performer or the Pilates Premier. These sturdy home machines begin at $200, with the average price about $300. Resources for Pilates' videotapes, home machines, and other Pilates equipment are Pilates Direct, 1-800-375-7520 or www.pilates-direct.com; QVC, 1-800-345-2525 or www.iqvc.com. Offering videotape sets is Collage Video, which stocks several dozen Pilates video workouts, www.collagevideo.com or call 1-800-433-6769 for a catalog or information.

What Works in Your Real World?

Let's now take all this advice and apply it to your "real world." First, can you set aside thirty to sixty minutes a day for alternating days of aerobic and strength-training workouts? If not, decide how much time you can devote to exercise. Set a specific goal. Then let's make sure you wisely use whatever time you can give to exercise to keep the most important aspects of fitness incorporated in your workout. I like this advice from fitness expert Kevin Makely:

Any exercise is better than nothing at all. However, if you're looking to increase your overall fitness, lose weight, or even increase muscle tone, you should always exercise intensely enough to work up a light sweat and get your heart beating at your personal training level.[14]

The most important thing to keep in your workout is the three-part approach to fitness—aerobic exercise, strength training, and stretching exercises. If you are doing some exercise now, take a look at your usual week and see if any of these three components are missing. Then add what you need to those you are already doing.

I would discourage you from investing large amounts of money in expensive gym memberships or costly home treadmills, elliptical machines, or weight machines unless you have tried them and are certain you will use them. A great resource for information on what brands and models of fitness machines may best meet your needs is *Consumer Reports* magazine, the March 2002 issue, in an article entitled "Stay Fit!" Also consider an inexpensive gym such as the YMCA, or effective yet low-priced home equipment—three- to five-pound barbells, low cost abdominal strengthening devices such as the Ab-Slide machine, large exercise balls, jump ropes, and exercise videos.

"What's an easy way to get more exercise on a busy schedule?"

It's Never Too Late to Start—If You Start Smart

As long as you are conscious, can still breathe, and have a beating heart, it's not too late to start exercising. Of course, you need to take appropriate care in your return to exercise. Consult your doctor if you are making a radical change in your activity level or if you recently had any medical problems or procedures that could affect your ability to exercise. As we will discuss in chapter 10, there often are painful consequences when you plunge into a rigorous exercise routine without taking your current level of fitness into account. These injuries can put you back on the sidelines for a long time.

Wearing the right shoes for the exercise you choose is another key to preventing injuries and discomfort. Do you need a shoe designed for walking? Or one designed for running? When you compare these shoes, you will see big differences in their construction that will protect you from heel and knee injuries.

Slowly warm up your muscles before beginning to exercise. You can do this simply by walking around a little and swinging your arms. Stretch your arms all the way up, all the way out in front, and out to each side. Begin your exercise activity at a less intense pace because the first minutes of exercise will do the best job of warming up your muscles.

For a long time, the belief has circulated that you must push yourself to as intense a level as is possible when you exercise. But moderate exercise is very effective—and much safer! In addition, we now know that you burn fat even if the workout is fewer than twenty minutes in length.

If you have not yet started to exercise, think of a way you can start to do the activity of your choice regularly—and ideal is three times a week for at least half an hour. Then take the first step. Maybe your first step will be to rent an exercise video to see if you like it, or to call your recreation department and find out what classes are offered or what team sports are available. Or maybe your step is making a jogging or walking date with a friend. Just discover what you love to do and start doing it. You will be so glad you did.

Part Two

Chart a Course That Protects Your Health

7

Pick the Doctors That Are Right for You

Your spa "package" includes expert advice on practical steps you can take to chart a course that protects your health. The first step is to choose health care providers you are confident will be in your corner when you need them. If you haven't already, now is the time to pick the doctors who are right for you. You need to choose a primary-care physician and a regular dentist, and most moms also need a separate ob-gyn doctor.

"Pick a doctor—any doctor." It sounds like a tableside magician about to do an amazing card trick. If only there were an all-knowing magician who could riffle through all the unfamiliar names on your insurance list and—*voilá!*—skillfully pull out the perfect match for you. Unfortunately, that magic trick isn't available, so we are left with the insurance-book list, which is a sea of unfamiliar doctors' names. How do you know whom to choose? When pressed for time, there is a temptation to choose a name that sounds nice or familiar. Ignore the temptation. You don't have to leave this decision up to chance or magic. If you stick to the following principles, choosing your health care team should be an easier process.

Know What to Look For

You probably put some time and effort into selecting the right pediatrician for your children, right? Well, you deserve the same treatment to find your physician. The right doctor will

- listen to your symptoms and concerns,
- answer your questions in a way you can understand,
- be covered by your insurance and use hospitals on your plan,
- schedule you for routine health exams and tests,
- see you in the office when you are acutely ill (without waiting two weeks),
- have a courteous staff, and
- be close enough to your home or work to make appointments convenient.

This is more than a wish list—you have the *right* to have a doctor who fits this bill. And although most doctors feel pressure to see many more patients each day than was common in years before (due to managed-care medicine), there *are* doctors everywhere who still give this level of service to their patients.

Many moms have ob-gyn doctors they are very happy with. In fact, some will try to use these physicians as their primary-care doctors. I advise you *not* to do this unless you specifically discuss this with your ob-gyn doctor and he or she agrees to take on this responsibility. While you probably are healthy now, if, for example, a heart problem or diabetes were to suddenly appear, your ob-gyn may not feel as comfortable managing your health problem as an internal medicine doctor or family practice physician would be.

Choose the right doctor before a health problem arises. Shopping for the right doctor when you are battling an illness or disease is very distressing. You may even be too ill to do such a search.

Other factors to consider are whether you prefer a male or female physician, and whether you prefer an older doctor with decades of experience or a younger doctor who may be more up-to-date on the latest treatments and theories in medicine but has fewer years of experience.

Also important to check is whether the doctor is "board certified," which means she has passed the exams specific to her special area of medicine (like internal medicine boards or family practice boards). Board certification gives you assurance that the doctor has the necessary credentials to be practicing medicine in a specific field of medicine. Usually the doctor's receptionist or nurse can verify this fact over the phone.

Know Where to Look

Ideally your doctor, whom you've known and loved for years, will be listed on the "Preferred Provider" insurance list year after year. But the reality is that insurance changes can leave us with a long list of unfamiliar names. So where do you go to find the new "Dr. Right"? Try the following measures:

Ask your previous primary-care or your ob-gyn doctor whom he or she recommends from your list. Many doctors will be happy to look at a copy of your list if you take or send it in. Also ask your favorite nurse whom they recommend. Nurses often have some of the best insight into choosing a "good" doctor. Ask a friend who lives in your area who her doctor is and whether she is happy with the care.

Ask your pastor if there is a doctor in the congregation that he or she would recommend. If you desire a Christian physician, you can contact the Christian Medical & Dental Associations to find out if any of the medical doctors or dentists on your list are also members of CMDA. Search online for a doctor in your area by logging on to www.cmdahome.org and typing in the "search" box the phrase: *Christian Doctor search.* Or contact CMDA by phone: 1-423-844-1000.

If you are still without a good lead, many cities (especially those with large hospitals) have physician referral services. You can find them in the yellow pages of your phone book or by calling a hospital.

Confirm That This Doctor Is Right for You

Now that you have one or more leads, it is time to have the right doctor *please* stand up. These steps will help you find out which of the recommended doctors fits your wish list. Most of them can be done over the phone:

- Call the office and speak to the receptionist to get a feel for how you might be treated on the phone.
- Verify whether this doctor is still on your insurance plan, whether he or she is board certified in his or her specialty, and what days and hours he or she is in the office.
- Ask how long it usually takes to get an appointment for a sick visit and a physical when you are well.
- Find out whether the doctor will allow you to come in and meet him or her before making your final choice (doctors often will do this over the phone instead).
- Have ready a question or two to ask the doctor. Avoid questions that require lengthy answers, since your visit will be brief. Pick instead questions that help you get a feel for whether this is a doctor with whom you will be comfortable.

Good questions to ask the doctor:

- If I call the office and wish to speak to you instead of a nurse, is that a problem?
- When could I expect that I would hear back from you?
- What do you think about patients taking vitamins and nutritional supplements?
- How many years have you been in practice?
- Do you plan to continue practicing in this area for many years?

Or use my personal favorite:

- Why should I choose you as my doctor?

Or the really tough one:

- Have you ever had a malpractice suit brought against you?

Even though your available time to do all this may be scarce, remember that the time you invest now in choosing the right doctor for yourself is well spent. It's hard to measure the value of peace of mind. But when you're faced with a serious health issue and have a doctor you like and know you can trust, you'll be glad you took the time. The peace of mind from that combination is priceless.

The Drill on Dentists and Dental Care

Most of the same principles you'll use to find the right doctor apply to finding the right dentist and dental office. You will likely be seeing both a dentist and a dental hygienist on a regular basis, so it's important that you feel comfortable with all the professionals in the office.

A dental checkup is something that many of us conveniently forget to schedule since dental checkups and cleanings are not the most pleasant ways to spend time. Once we have put it off, we are more likely to put it off again. Then we become embarrassed and it becomes even harder to go back and "face the music."

But there are many important reasons to get over the past and get back on an every-six-months checkup plan. I consulted one of the best dentists for you on this matter, Talmadge Carter, D.D.S., my father.[1]

"Regular dental checkups are like regular oil changes. It's much less expensive and less invasive to have a checkup regularly than to have to rebuild your engine, or in this case your mouth," says Dr. Tal Carter. "Initially, checkups should be every six months. Then your dentist can determine if your needs are for more or less frequent visits. Each individual has a different system, so some need cleanings as often as every three months. If your dentist reevaluates you after that initial six-month visit, he or she can advise you whether you require every three-month, six-month, or even once-a-year visits."

Dr. Carter has some special advice for moms who are expecting: "During pregnancy hormonal changes reflect in the tissues of the mouth. This can promote gingivitis and swelling of the gums and can lead to gum recession and bone resorbtion if you do not take proper care. As soon as you know you are pregnant, you should have a good, thorough cleaning to remove any irritants that can cause gum irritation. But make certain you have no X rays until preferably after the baby is delivered. In an emergency situation, if you need to have an X ray, be sure you request double lead aprons with a thyroid collar for extra protection."

For daily dental care, Dr. Carter recommends "brushing with a soft toothbrush, preferably within ten to fifteen minutes after every meal, because that's when the bacteria eat *their* meal, producing an acid that causes cavities. If you cannot brush, at least swish and swallow with water to remove the food debris, bacteria, and acid. Massage your gums with a soft toothbrush each day, and floss at least every evening. Glide is the floss I strongly recommend." He also recommends you get instructions from your dentist or hygienist on the correct way to floss.

Many moms wonder about the numerous electric and sonic toothbrushes on the market now. According to many dental experts, *any* mechanical toothbrush is superior to hand brushing. Another worthy device to consider is the old standard, the WaterPik. As Dr. Carter puts it, "it hoses down your teeth like hosing down a sidewalk and removes debris from all the crevices."

Become Aware of Your Dental Inheritance

Depending on our family histories, some of us do inherit the tendency toward cavity-prone teeth or gum disease, or both. But proper dental care and regular checkups can minimize these risks. Having a dentist you feel comfortable with will make going to these routine checkups much less daunting, so don't put off finding the right dentist.

Now that you have your doctors and your dentist lined up, and know how to minimize the risks from your dental inheritance, we'll talk about your medical inheritance in the next chapter and how you can reduce your risks with screening tests and other healthy choices.

8

Inherited Disease Risks and Screening Tests

We get more than blue or brown eyes and straight or curly hair from the beloved family members who came before us. We inherit health risks. What health risks run in your family? Some families are more likely to develop heart disease; some develop diabetes; other families have many members who develop cancer. But the good news is that if we make wise lifestyle choices, follow sound medical advice, and screen for these diseases, we can stall or avoid all together developing these medical conditions.

The bad news, however, is that some people, no matter how much they do that is right, will *still* develop serious medical conditions. I am deeply disturbed as both a physician and a Christian when I hear anyone say that God wants all of us to be healthy all the time, and that as long as we are living according to his laws, we will be healthy. If a person is ill, these folks say it is because he or she is breaking some of God's laws for living. This is one of the most damaging attitudes for an ill person to encounter. Floods of guilt and despair engulf an already weakened person. This attitude is *not* based on the Bible or on medical science.

Look at Job, for example. He was the godliest of men in his time, yet God allowed him to be plagued by countless calamities (Job 1:8–12;

2:3–7). And remember the apostle Paul, who prayed "three times" that his physical ailment would go away. But God did not cure his ailment, and instead answered, "My grace is sufficient for you, for my power is made perfect in weakness" (2 Corinthians 12:7–10).

I believe God gave each of us a measure of health that is our job to protect. Some are given more health for their lifetime and others are given a sparser measure. God made us that way, and unless he chooses to heal one who becomes ill, that person may remain ill *despite* living by God's laws. Sometimes it is God's will *not* to heal. Yet that person can live with the assurance that God's grace is sufficient for her.

Keeping this in mind, let's focus on what we *can* do to limit our development of medical illnesses. It has been proven that the following factors often push your risks into the reality of medical illness:

- smoking
- alcohol abuse
- diet high in saturated fats
- chronically high stress load

If your lifestyle includes one or more of these factors, you are *asking* for health trouble. But it is your choice whether you include or exclude these risk factors—and today you can begin to exclude any that affect your life.

It's Not Too Early to Think about These Diseases

In the MOPS Moms Health Survey, the majority of women ranked heart disease, stroke, and diabetes all very low on their list of health concerns. That's not surprising since most moms surveyed were between the ages of twenty-three and forty-two (with one sixty-two-year-old surveyed). But I hope to show you that the health choices you make now—in your twenties, thirties, and early forties—can dramatically affect whether you are dealing with these diseases in your forties, fifties, sixties, and beyond. These conditions are not reserved solely for women in their midlife and beyond. Some of you may face them much sooner. That is why knowing what to look for and having routine screening tests are so important to your health.

Signs You Must Not Ignore

Coronary heart disease starts out as the third leading cause of death for women ages twenty-five to forty-four, climbs to the second leading cause of death for women ages forty-five to sixty-four, and then becomes the leading cause of death in women over sixty-five. That may not surprise you. But a statistic that may surprise you is that heart disease and stroke kill nearly ten times as many women each year as breast cancer does.[1] Did you know that in every year since 1984, cardiovascular disease has claimed the lives of more females than males?[2] Plus, 63 percent of the women who die suddenly from heart disease had no previous symptoms of heart disease.[3] So it is clear that we must look for signs of heart disease in women long before we expect to find any.

> *"Could I have a heart attack at my age, 30?"*

According to many experts, one of the main reasons women die more often with their first attack is because the symptoms of a woman's heart attack may differ greatly from what we expect. The classic symptoms of a man's heart attack are well known: crushing pain in the mid-chest, pain radiating up to the neck or down the left arm, anxiety, and sweating. But women may have symptoms such as unusual fatigue, unusual or new shortness of breath during little or no activity, dizziness, lower chest pressure or discomfort, back pain, nausea, or upper abdominal discomfort or pressure.[4]

Weight Loss You Didn't Bargain For

Although most women think unexpected weight loss would be like a gift from heaven, from a health standpoint it is a red flag that says something may be wrong. Your weight loss, we hope, may just mean that new, healthy eating habits and increased exercise are paying off. But if you have made no lifestyle changes that could explain your smaller pants' size, your doctor needs to see you to check for conditions such as a possible infection in your system, abnormal hormone levels, diabetes, cancer, or even the effects of severe stress. So if you suddenly are, for no known reason, the "incredible shrinking woman," make an appointment with your doctor immediately for an exam and any appropriate tests. Finding a problem early means proper treatment closer to the beginning of an illness and a better chance for a full recovery.

> *"What medical tests are absolutely necessary to ensure good health?"*

Screening Tests (see chart at end of chapter)

Why screen? Because doctors can catch early stages of many forms of cancer, coronary heart disease, diabetes, and some forms of kidney disease, then stop the disease, or at least the progression, in many cases. Yet, according to a government study, more than 50 percent of all Americans do not get the screening and preventive health care that is recommended.[5]

So let's be trendsetters and change that statistic. First, schedule an annual health exam. An easy way to remember when to schedule your annual screening is to use your birthday as a reminder.

Cholesterol Testing

In the MOPS Moms survey, cholesterol was the eighth most common topic that moms asked questions about. I'm glad you're asking about it because cholesterol blood levels are the most important aid we have for assessing your risk of having a heart attack. The different cholesterol levels (LDL, HDL, and total cholesterol) give us insight into the health of your arteries and, specifically, whether you have atherosclerosis (clogging and hardening of your arteries). Some people have inherited disorders that cause their cholesterol to be very high even if their diets are healthy and they are young. Unfortunately, too many of these folks find out about their risk too late and suffer a fatal first heart attack around the age of forty. This is why knowing your family history and getting screening tests regularly are both so important.

In 2001, new guidelines were established for screening cholesterol levels. All adults twenty years or older should have a "fasting lipoprotein panel" every five years (no food for nine to twelve hours prior to the test). This screening test measures LDL, HDL, total cholesterol, and triglyceride levels. If any of the levels are in the abnormal range, you need a retest every year.

"How often should my cholesterol level be checked?"

There are also new, stricter limits for what values are considered normal. Normal LDL = 100 mg/dl; cholesterol-lowering drugs and lifestyle changes are recommended if LDL is over 130 mg/dl. Normal HDL = between 40 and 60 mg/dl. Normal total cholesterol = less than 200. Normal triglycerides = less than 150 mg/dl.

Annual Blood Pressure Check

All women need their blood pressure checked each time they go to the doctor. Hypertension—or high blood pressure—strains the heart and blood vessels of the body, which increases the risk of both heart attack and stroke. In fact, high blood pressure is the risk factor most closely connected to an increased risk of stroke.[6] Yet hypertension usually has no clear physical signs to alert you that there is a problem.

Check for Diabetes

Diabetes is diagnosed by finding a high blood sugar level or sugar in the urine. There are also more sophisticated tests your doctor might order if one of these is abnormal. Several sources recommend having a blood sugar test every three years after age forty-five, but most experts look for it only if you have other risk factors, such as a family history of diabetes or obesity. If you are concerned or have any of these risk factors, when your doctor orders your fasting lipid panel (cholesterol test), ask for a fasting blood sugar test to be added.

Cancer Checkups

The American Cancer Society recommends a cancer-related checkup every three years for people ages twenty to forty and every year for those age forty and older.[7] The statistics about cancer can be frightening, but if you follow the recommended guidelines for cancer screening, even if you develop cancer, over 90 percent of cancers detected early can be cured. The ten most common types of cancer that affect women are (1) breast, (2) lung, (3) colon and rectum, (4) uterus, (5) non-Hodgkin's lymphoma, (6) melanoma of skin, (7) ovary, (8) thyroid, (9) pancreas, and (10) urinary bladder.[8]

To Mammogram or Not to Mammogram . . . That Is Now the Question

The standard in women's health was to start getting yearly mammograms once we reached the age of forty or sooner if there was a history of breast cancer in the family. It was a standard procedure because multiple research studies had shown that mammogram screening was finding large numbers of cases of breast cancer at a much earlier stage. One study showed a 30 percent decrease in the risk of dying from breast cancer in women who had been screened. Then in 2001 a study from Denmark brought this practice into question. The Danish researchers reported finding flaws in seven previous studies and suggested that there may not be enough reliable evidence to say that mammograms do more good than the potential harm caused by the radiation.

What symptoms should you look for? Early warning signs of cancer include:[9]

- A thickening or lump, in your breast or elsewhere, that is usually not painful
- Hoarseness or nagging cough
- Change in bowel habits
- Difficulty swallowing or indigestion
- Unusual bleeding or discharge
- A sore that does not heal
- Obvious change in a mole or wart
- Weight loss and loss of appetite
- Change in bladder habits

What do the rest of the experts say now? The American Cancer Society still *strongly* recommends that women continue to obtain mammograms every year after they turn forty. The National Cancer Institute recommends mammograms every one to two years after age forty. One of the reasons behind these recommendations for continuing mammograms is that the death rate from breast cancer slowly but surely decreased in the 1990s. The rate at which later-stage tumors were diagnosed also decreased because the cancers were being found earlier with the routine of an annual mammogram starting at age forty. Everyone would prefer to find a lower risk, low cost, alternative screening test to replace the mammogram, but that alternative has not yet been found. I side with the American Cancer Society, the National Cancer Institute, and the several other ob-gyn physicians that I consulted. Keep getting those mammograms, preferably every year, but at least every one to two years after your fortieth birthday. With about 200,000 new cases of breast cancer expected to be diagnosed this year, and about 40,000 women expected to die from breast cancer this year, I want to help keep you from becoming one of those statistics.[10]

This emphasis on mammograms does not minimize the importance of the exam you can do yourself: your monthly self breast exam. You will find an irregularity sooner and more easily than your doctor if you do the exam each month. The exam is best done at the end of your period, when your breasts are less likely to be sore. Make it a habit to do your self breast exam every month on the last day of your period. You can check them in the shower, in front of a mirror while standing, or reclined on your back. Start at the center of the breast and press in with your fingers, feeling for anything that feels like a hard, dried pea. Move outward with your fingers, like on a spoke of a bicycle wheel. Then move to the next spot and repeat. Move in a circular pattern, like going from one hour mark on a clock to the next hour mark. Notice any changes or thickenings that you haven't felt before. Be sure to check the large portion of each breast that is tucked under your armpit. Do this exam on both breasts each month, for it is one of the easiest things you can do to decrease your risk of fatal cancer.

Annual Pelvic Exam and Pap Test

The risk of getting cervical cancer sometime in your lifetime is 1 in 117. But this is a big improvement. Since the 1970s, the incidence and death rates from cancer of the cervix (the opening to the uterus, or womb) have dropped 40 percent.[11] That improvement is largely due to early detection by annual Pap smears, which can detect abnormal cells. All women eighteen and over should continue to have an annual pelvic exam and Pap test.

Colon Cancer Checks

Since colorectal cancer is the third leading cause of cancer deaths in women,[12] starting at age fifty, women should have the following tests: a yearly fecal occult blood test (tests for blood in your stool) and a flexible sigmoidoscopy test every five years. Other options are a double-contrast barium enema every five years or a colonoscopy every ten years. (All positive tests should be followed up with colonoscopy.)

Optional Screening Tests

Several other tests are optional, and you may wish to discuss them with your doctor. Urinalysis is a quick way to screen for many things that can go wrong in the body, including certain kidney problems and diabetes. A thyroid panel of tests might be indicated if you have extreme fatigue (to rule out low thyroid) or other symptoms that may indicate high thyroid levels. A complete blood count (CBC) tells if you are anemic ("iron poor blood") and is a basic screen for signs of infection and other blood disorders. Hearing, vision, and glaucoma screening usually are not recommended as routine tests until a woman is over fifty, but if you notice any decrease in your vision or hearing, contact your doctor.

Immunizations You Must Not Forget

Tetanus boosters need to be given every ten years. However, if you step on a rusty nail or are cut by an old rusted object between five to ten years after your last booster, you may wish to renew it at that time. I also recommend you have an influenza vaccine every year.

Skin Screening

Your skin is one of the most important areas of your body to examine regularly because it is exposed to so much every day. We will look at skin screening and skin care in detail in the next chapter as we continue charting the best course that will protect your health.

Schedule of Basic Screening Tests
for Every Mom

Screening Test	How Often	Starting When
Fasting Cholesterol / Lipid Panel	Every 5 years	Women over 20
Blood Pressure	Every year	Women over 18
Fasting Blood Glucose	Every 3 years	Women over 45 (or if at risk)
Mammogram	Every 1-2 years	Women over 40
Pelvic Exam and Pap Smear	Every year	Women over 18
Fecal Occult Blood Test	Every year	Women over 18
Flexible Sigmoidoscopy	Every 5 years	Women over 50
Colonoscopy	Every 10 years	Women over 50

9

Skin Care That Makes a Difference

Welcome to the skin care center of the MOPS Health Spa. Here we not only pamper your skin but evaluate it and educate you about skin care that can make a difference. So sit back and enjoy the relaxing music.

Beautiful skin. Isn't that what we all want? I'll let you in on the secret behind beautiful skin—when you have beautiful skin it is because you have healthy skin. There are some skin care basics we all need to follow, and not only because we want our skin to look as nice as possible for as long as possible. Skin is one of the most vulnerable parts of our body, and not guarding it can result in far worse consequences than wrinkles. It can result in death by melanoma.

Here Comes the Sun

The one thing you could do that would not only protect your skin to the maximum but also keep it looking younger longer would be to avoid exposure to the sun (and sunlamps and tanning beds). The sun is your skin's worst enemy! And it's not enough to avoid baking in the sun while trying to get a tan; you also need to be aware of all the other times you receive a hefty dose of sun exposure when you may not even realize it. How often have you diligently covered your children with sunscreen but it slipped your mind to coat your skin as well? Every fifteen minutes here and fifteen minutes there of sun exposure adds up to a lot of sun damage over the years. That is why it is best to work the use of sunscreen into your daily routine. Many facial moisturizers now have sunscreen incorporated into the product. However, you need to check the strength of sunscreen used (it should be SPF 15 or higher), and whether it protects against both UV-A (the deeply penetrating aging rays) and UV-B rays (the superficial sunburning rays)—both of which are very damaging.

Run from the Sun

Beware of the false sense of security many feel who go outdoors wearing sunscreen and think they are now safe in the sun. Recent studies show an increase in skin cancer rates in some sunscreen wearers, although other studies do not make this association.[1] It does make you wonder if some of these folks with skin cancer spent more time in the sun than was sensible *because* they were wearing sunscreen. Sunscreen is only a screen; it's not a cloak capable of blocking you from all the sun's rays. So even with sunscreen you will get some sun damage over time. The best answer is to *block* your skin from the sun with clothing, or avoid exposure altogether during the peak hours of sun intensity, from 10 A.M. to 4 P.M. Avoid tanning beds, since they may be more harmful to your skin than regular sun exposure. The best attitude toward tanning is *the best tan is a fake tan.*

Fashionable and Wise Sun Attire

Dress like a movie star going incognito when you are out in the sun. Don a three-inch-wide brimmed hat (or one that also has a flap over the back of your neck), and UV-blocking sunglasses with large lenses (to decrease the development of cataracts). Clothing is a helpful screen if it covers most of your skin and if the fabric has a tight weave and is a darker color that absorbs UV rays. Ideally, clothing should cover you with long sleeves and pant legs, and there should be a collar to protect your neck. Now, I know it sounds ridiculous to wear dark colored clothing with long sleeves and long pants in the middle of a hot, summer day. But at least consider it if you are very sensitive to the sun or have a family history of skin cancer. Another option is to try one of the lines of sun-protective clothing, like Solumbria.[2] These products are made from patented sun protective fabrics.

The Scoop on Sunscreen

Qualifications and Quantity Both *Matter*

It isn't enough that your sunscreen has a minimum SPF (Sun Protection Factor) of 15. I recommend an SPF of 40, and make sure the sunscreen works against both UV-A and UV-B rays (check the label). The amount of sunscreen you apply matters a lot if you want the promised degree of protection. If you are like most people, you probably are not using enough to truly protect yourself. This is not a time to be stingy and frugal. Doctors recommend one palmful (about one ounce) of sunscreen per application for most adults. So if you have a four-ounce tube of sunscreen, it should not last beyond four outings. So gob on the sunscreen, because it can't help you if you don't apply enough. And at the end of the season, discard leftover sunscreen. Some people break out in a skin rash from using old sunscreen. Do you want a "super sunscreen"? Then get sunscreen containing titanium dioxide or zinc oxide, and consider those with avobenzone (also known as Parsol 1789).[3]

> *Remember, your lips need TLC and protection too, so use lip balm with an SPF of 15 regularly.*

The Best Time for Sunscreen

When you apply sunscreen greatly affects how well it works. After applying sunscreen, it takes at least twenty to thirty minutes for the protective ingredients in your sunscreen to activate protection in your skin cells. Unless you apply it thirty minutes before going out, you will likely spend the first thirty minutes outside getting sunburned while you apply sunscreen and before it becomes active. But wait, there is more. After spending several hours in the sun, especially after you have been in the water, reapply your sunscreen even if you are using a waterproof product.

One of the best waterproof sunscreens is waterproof regular Bull Frog brand. Bull Frog is the perfect name for this product, because once it is on it feels like you have an amphibious outer layer. It really works well. Apply according to the label's instructions: Before going out, apply one layer to all exposed skin. Then apply a second layer on top. Reapply after being in the water.

Medications That Can Make Your Skin Fry

Certain medications can dramatically increase your tendency to burn in the sun, even when you wear sunscreen. So take extra care if you are on these or any other drugs said to increase your sensitivity to the sun:

- Antibiotics like tetracycline, minocycline, doxycycline, ciprofloxacin, and sulfa drugs
- Retin-A topical cream or gel
- Diuretics like hydrochlorothiazide
- Oral contraceptives such as mircette

Nutrition That Can Decrease Sun Damage

We now know about Bugs Bunny's secret sunscreen, and you can use it too! Recent antioxidant research suggests that taking in carotenoids (as in carrots, "doc") and other antioxidants may help protect you from sun damage, providing an internal sunscreen. The best way to get these antioxidants is by eating lots of fruits and vegetables, but research has also looked at nutritional supplements. One study looked at patient skin reactions to twelve weeks of UV light exposure while on a supplement of either 25 mg carotenes a day or 25 mg carotenes plus 500 IU vitamin E a day. Both groups had significant protection from sunburn, but the group getting carotenes plus vitamin E did better.[4] Other studies suggest vitamin E with vitamin C (500–1,000 mg a day), or selenium (50–200 mcg) help. These are not to be relied on in place of topical sunscreen. Consider them only as an added help.

Sunburn, Skin Cancer, and Statistics

Did you know that skin cancer is the most common cancer in the United States, with more than 1 million new cases diagnosed each year? According to the American Cancer Society, women under the age of forty are the fastest growing group of skin cancer patients. Yikes! You may also be surprised to learn that even one peeling sunburn before the age of eighteen can double your lifetime risk of getting melanoma. It is estimated that 23,500 women in the U.S. will be diagnosed with melanoma in 2002, and six of every seven deaths from skin cancer are from melanoma.[5] It is clear that we need to pay attention to our sun exposure. When it comes to sun exposure and sun damage, it all adds up.

There are three types of skin cancer: basal cell, squamous cell, and deadly malignant melanoma.

Risk Factors for Skin Cancer

In addition to the factor of your lifetime amount of exposure, there are skin cancer risk factors that you cannot control, such as the increased risk if you are fair skinned, freckle easily, are blonde or red-haired, or have blue or green eyes. Skin cancer (especially melanoma) also tends to run in families. It also depends on where you live. If you live in the high mountains, in the desert, or near the equator, your UV exposure will be greater.

Danger Signs

With all this bad news about skin cancer, there is one bit of good news; *all* skin cancers can be successfully treated if they are discovered and treated early. Therefore, your best defense (other than avoiding sun exposure) is to screen your skin for suspicious changes every month.

Signs of skin damage are freckles, a tan, wrinkles, sunburn, cataracts, and ultimately, skin cancer. But what does skin cancer look like? It can be:[6]

1. A scaly red spot
2. A change in the color, shape, or size of a mole
3. Bleeding in a mole or other growth
4. Any new skin growth

Teach Your Moles the "A-B-C-Ds"

Do you have a lot of moles? A family history of skin cancer? Then you must screen your moles for changes every month. It's as easy as looking for:

- Asymmetry (left side not like the right side)
- Border irregularity
- Color variation (lesion not all of the same color)
- Diameter (larger than 6 millimeters, which is the size of pencil eraser)

Melanomas usually have these changes.

The Skinny on Skin Care

From "How do you treat wrinkles and age spots?" to "How can I clear my acne?" the moms in our survey had many questions about effective skin care. I brought in two consultants that you will meet very shortly, but first let's tackle the bumpy issue of acne in adult moms.[7]

Acne—at My Age?

The American Academy of Dermatology estimates that more than 12 million American adults are battling with acne, with women affected four times more often than men. This gender difference is one of the reasons hormonal shifts are blamed for a lot of adult acne. Stress and genetic tendency also are big factors in triggering adult acne. But for the most part, dirt and foods eaten do not play a big role. Acne is caused when pores become clogged and then infected. To decrease your chances of developing acne or triggering flare-ups, gently wash your face twice a day (never go to sleep with your makeup still on), and use non-comedogenic facial creams and products (especially avoid mineral oil found in many foundations and face powders). "Comedogenic" means it may cause comedones, which are clogged pores, or commonly known as pimples.

What if despite your best efforts you end up with acne—then what? The over-the-counter approaches usually utilize either a base of benzoyl peroxide (like Proactiv brand) or salicylic acid (like Philosophy brand acne-care products) to treat the blemishes and help prevent new ones. Although you need a certain amount of "drying effect" to help clear blemishes, a big mistake is letting the skin become overly dried out because then the skin thinks you need *more oil* and pumps it out to the surface. So be sure to moisturize with a light non-comedogenic product morning and night.

If your over-the-counter efforts do not succeed, see your doctor or a dermatologist for additional treatment options. One is a topical antibiotic product (like erythromycin gel). If that is not successful, then you may go to an oral antibiotic. If still more help is needed, Retin-A is a good step. With all of these treatments you need to be patient with results. It can take four to eight weeks for the full effect to appear. Many women find their acne improves on oral contraceptives, so your doctor may also suggest these. In very rare situations, a last step may be the drug Accutane (but Accutane can cause birth defects, so you must never become pregnant while on Accutane).

The last words on acne are, don't pick or pop your zits. I know it is so tempting, but both of these actions usually cause further skin damage and can leave permanent scars.

Dr. D's Top Picks for Over-the-Counter, Low-Cost Skin Care Products

Now for our first consultant: We are fortunate to have with us a dermatologist, Dr. Zoe Draelos, who is Clinical Associate Professor of Dermatology at Wake Forest University School of Medicine and a researcher who has published extensively on cosmetic products.

"I would recommend the following products for busy moms. I have selected these products because they are available nationwide in mass merchandisers, grocery stores, and drugstores. They offer excellent technology for the cost, which is a good economic value for the woman who wants value and efficacy in her skin care."

- Gentle facial cleanser: *Olay Foaming Face Wash for Sensitive Skin*
- Good body, face, and eyelid moisturizer: *Cetaphil cream*
- Good hand and foot moisturizer: *Neutrogena Norwegian Formula Hand Cream*
- Good facial sunscreen and moisturizer: *Olay Complete SPF15*
- Good body cleanser for rough, dry skin: *Olay Complete Body Wash for Dry Skin*
- Good sunscreen for outdoor activities: *Neutrogena Sensitive Skin Sunscreen*
- Good water resistant sunscreen for children: *Bull Frog Face Gel and Body Gel*
- Good nighttime exfoliant cleaning with good cosmetic removal: *Olay Daily Facials for Sensitive Skin*

How to Keep Your Skin Looking Young

We also are privileged to have with us Bill Dascombe, M.D., a plastic surgeon who also has a background in skin research and an extensive skin care practice in Savannah, Georgia. He will share with us what does and doesn't help when it comes to treating aging skin.

Q: ***What is the best approach to battle the changes in a woman's skin as she ages?***

Dr. Dascombe: "Spend five minutes in the morning and five minutes at night on your skin. By investing a little bit of time each day with the right products, you will preserve the beauty and health of your skin."

Q: ***What is the safest and most effective way to combat wrinkles as they appear?***

Dr. Dascombe: "If there was any one single agent for women to use on their skin, I would suggest Retin-A. It is by far the most effective agent to combat wrinkles. Retin-A helps to build collagen, the scaffolding of the skin. Loss of collagen and another substance, elastin, are what causes wrinkles.

"There are varying concentrations and formulations of Retin-A, and this prescription should be used under the care of a physician. It is safe and can be used long-term without complications. The strength of Retin-A that I recommend is 0.05 percent to start. You may need to work up to 0.1 percent. If you have dry or sensitive skin, it is best in a base called renova, while if you have oily skin, use 0.05 percent in gel or cream base. Another good form is Retin-A Micro, which is a timed-release formulation and 0.1 percent.

> *"What is the best over-the-counter skin care for aging skin?"*

"It is best used as a part of a skin care program and not by itself alone. I have tried over ten of the top medical grade skin care programs in the United States. I favor Obagi.[8] (I have no financial interest in the company.) Obagi is a Retin-A based program that was developed by a

California dermatologist, Dr. Obagi. I like it because I find it meets the skin care needs of 95 percent of people, based on age, race, and skin type. And 95 to 96 percent of my patients love it. Obagi is a medically supervised skin care program that you can get from your doctor. (Some of the Obagi products can be purchased at www.drugstore.com.) It works out to about $100 per month for the first six months, with a maintenance program of $50 per month. It is an investment that pays for itself if a woman is buying a lot of makeup, etc., because a majority of women report that they stop using makeup."

Q: What about the following treatments?

Micropeel/Microdermabrasion with sugars

Dr. Dascombe: "This polishes the outside layer of the skin and makes the skin look and feel better. It doesn't affect the deeper layers of the skin. If you can tolerate Retin-A, this cream is a better investment of your hard-earned money."

Alpha-hydroxy acids

Dr. Dascombe: "Alpha- and beta-hydroxy acids are very mild skin treatments. They sometimes help women with mild acne and give mild improvement in the texture and tone of the skin. They do not affect the deeper layers of the skin."

Topical Vitamin C

Dr. Dascombe: "Topical vitamin C formulations are getting better and better. They serve as an antioxidant and slowly help to build collagen, the scaffolding of the skin. They are used wonderfully in conjunction with Retin-A. Ten percent Vitamin C concentration is the industry norm. It is very unstable so when it is exposed to air it loses its potency, but if the bottle is used up within six months it is not likely to be a problem."

Topical collagen-containing creams

Dr. Dascombe: "Stay away from them. They smell lovely and feel great, but they don't do much for the health and longevity of the skin."

Dr. Dascombe also recommends daily facial sunscreen in the SPF 30–40 range. However, he does not recommend higher than SPF 40 because there can be irritation of the skin from chemicals.

Remember, moms, the best way to keep that sunny glow is to keep your skin as far from the sun's damaging rays as possible.

10

Physical Injury—An Occupational Hazard for Moms

Did you know that carrying a diaper bag or purse can be hazardous to your health? Especially when you add to that a forty-pound kiddo on your hip. If you are like nearly all of us when we were first-time moms you pack every conceivable object you might need for the next month into your new suitcase-sized diaper bag "just in case." You sling it over one shoulder, then pick up your baby in the carrier and start out. My back hurts just reminiscing about those overloaded days!

The most recent statistics show that over 36 percent of new moms are over the age of thirty.[1] With so many moms now starting their families in their thirties and older, there is a greater risk that they will sustain injuries just doing what they have to do as moms. But it isn't just new moms who are at risk; *all* moms are. And the occupational hazards of parenting change as your children grow. So whether it is carrying around an infant and all the hardware that comes with them or lifting and toting around your toddler or preschooler, your physical body is at great risk.

These physical health risks include neck and back strain and muscle imbalances set up by frequently toting heavy bags on one shoulder or your child on your hip. Add to that all sorts of other sprains, strains, and ligament and tendon injuries. All these can come from the busy life of keeping up with a busy child.

Uplifting Advice on Back Pain

To give you the best advice on how to prevent these injuries and treat them once they happen, I consulted Steven Copp, M.D., head of the Division of Orthopedics at Scripps Clinic of San Diego.[2] Dr. Copp is an orthopedic physician and surgeon who sees a lot of moms and dads whose bodies have taken a beating while caring for their kids.

> *"How can I relieve this constant lower back pain?"*

According to Dr. Copp, the most common of these injuries is back strain, which results in acute (or short-term) lower back pain. Lower back pain in parents is most commonly caused by their poor lifting techniques—not only of the child but also all the hardware involved, such as strollers and car seats. Dr. Copp says these injuries especially show up in those older parents who have poor lifting techniques. The strain on the back may aggravate early degenerative changes in the back and lead to pain.

The most significant strain on the disks and muscles of the spine happens when parents try to lift a load that is not close to their body. An example is when moms lift children out of cribs using outstretched arms. The second type of lifting that is most potentially damaging is lifting and turning with a load extended from you, such as when a mom bends over and twists to assist a sometimes struggling child in or out of the car seat in the backseat of a two-door car.

So what is the right way to lift? First you need to get a realistic view of what you are lifting, realizing what you have become accustomed to lifting. It is very easy to lift our children at birth since most weigh six to nine pounds. But very quickly you are lifting a load of thirty to fifty pounds.

Here is the proper way to lift your precious cargo:

1. Bend your knees before you lift.
2. Lift with your hands and arms as close to you as possible, and with a straight back.
3. Use your abdominal muscles to take the strain off your back and to support it as you lift.
4. Have toddlers and preschoolers help by standing up in the crib before you pick them up, and teach them to *gently* move upward when you say "up."

So what do you do if you strain your back and find yourself with lower back pain? Most back pain is acute, or short-term. Dr. Copp recommends:

- Anti-inflammatory medication—usually for about two weeks if this is acute pain. If chronic, then it is used as long-term pain management. This category includes over-the-counter choices like ibuprofen (Advil) and naprosyn (Aleve), but also many effective prescription choices. Check with your doctor to verify that your anti-inflammatory medicine is safe to take if you are pregnant or nursing.
- Education—about how this happened in the first place and how with proper lifting techniques you may prevent recurrences. Also, it is important to understand that the back cannot heal if a mom continues to lift during the recovery period and reinjures herself.
- Return to a better level of fitness—through a walking program for forty minutes a day, and back and abdominal strengthening exercises.
- If needed, physical therapy may help.

Bed Rest or No Bed Rest?

Should moms go to bed and avoid movement when there is low back pain? Or should they lightly exercise? Dr. Copp says that walking around and standing are not harmful activities, but prolonged sitting may strain the back so it is not advised. Of course, there should be no lifting until the acute back pain is better. Many studies show that light exercise may be effective in helping you recover from many common back injuries.[3] But this assumes that you follow the doctor's advice and don't reinjure yourself by overdoing or doing heavy lifting during this time of recovery. Ask for and accept help until your injury is healed. Then be smart about body mechanics.

The good news for acute back pain sufferers is that "85 percent are better in two weeks, 90 percent are better in four weeks, and 95 percent are better in six," says Dr. Copp.

Chiropractor Care? Acupuncture?

There definitely is a place in back-pain treatment for both chiropractic and acupuncture therapies. Dr. Copp says, "There is evidence in the medical literature that chiropractic care can shorten the duration of back pain if it is acute in onset."[4] Researchers also found that chiropractic care does not seem to help much with chronic back pain.[5] The long-term treatment for chronic back pain includes lifestyle modifications, improving one's fitness, and physical therapy.

Acupuncture may be best utilized if a mom has chronic pain. It does not appear to be of much help for those with acute pain.

Sprains, Strains, and All the Other Injuries

The second most common parent injury, according to Dr. Copp, is a painful condition called *DeQuervain's tenosynovitis* of the tendons of the thumb. This condition results from poor lifting technique and repetitive motions like grasping, squeezing, and wringing. Moms with this have pain on the side of their wrist just above the thumb. If not treated, the pain may spread up the forearm or down into the thumb. The usual treatment is to first try to decrease the repetitive motions and keep the wrist in natural alignment by wearing a splint or brace for a short time to rest the tendons and quiet the inflammation. Anti-inflammatory medications are also used (again, such as OTC ibuprofen and naprosyn, and prescription choices). Usually these measures take care of the problem. If not, then other options such as surgery would be considered.[6]

A myriad of other physical injuries are often incurred when carrying and caring for children. Especially when playing with children. Many a mom sprains her ankle, injures her knee, pulls muscles, and tears tendons—all in the name of loving her child.

Remember the word *RICE* so you know what to do if injured:

- Rest your injury for at least twenty-four to forty-eight hours, which means use crutches and do not bear weight on it.
- Ice the injured part for twenty minutes at a time, the sooner the better and several times a day.
- Compression—wrap the injured part with an ace bandage.
- Elevate the injured part, keeping it higher than the heart.

If it is clear that the injury is more serious, contact your doctor to see if you should be seen in the office or elsewhere, such as by an orthopedist or at the emergency room.

Tips to Help Prevent Muscle Imbalances

Next, let's revisit the issue of your heavy diaper bag or purse, along with the child you always carry on the same hip.

- Rethink what you really need to carry in a purse or diaper/tote bag.
- Choose the smallest bag possible (if it's big it has the magnetic tendency to attract more and more items, and then you are once again bent over walking like Quasimodo).

- Stash what you can in the car. Keep a big "master bag" in the car and take out only the items you need when out and about. This way you aren't carrying half your child's toys or clothing.
- Switch off which side you carry your child on.
- Pilates exercises stretch and relieve fatigue and stress; they also strengthen your body symmetrically. Research confirms that Pilates not only helps prevent injuries but it also has been shown to help rehabilitate those with back pain, muscle imbalances, and other injuries.[7]

Be Smart about Your Level of Fitness

More than a few times I've had limping parents—and others wearing slings—bring in their children, who look better than their parents. The conversation usually starts something like this: "Well, I hadn't done a cartwheel in twenty years . . ." or "I wanted to show him how to swing on the bars at the playground." It is hard to face, but be realistic about your current level of physical fitness before throwing your back or shoulder out with a cartwheel or an Olympic attempt on the parallel bars. You usually *can* improve your level of fitness if it is not what it used to be. And Pilates is a great way to start, since it is a workout that strengthens the whole body. You can easily adjust the level of difficulty to what you need.

Oops! I Did It Again

Once you've become injured, one of the biggest issues is preventing a reinjury while you are healing. Reinjury is often the case with back injuries and limb sprains because it is so hard to not use your back and limbs, especially when you are caring for young children. There is no magic solution to this dilemma. Just try harder to not do what you know you should not do while you are healing. Otherwise it will take even longer to heal, or worse, you could develop a chronic problem.

Home Accident Prevention

Accident-proofing your home isn't just for your child's safety—it's also for yours. Most parents are quick to baby-proof and child-proof their homes to protect their child from preventable accidents. But what about your safety? You need to do some parent-proofing on a regular basis. Watch out for toys left on the floor that can trip you and cause falls. Beware when you are multitasking—doing many things at once; you are more likely to be injured. The same goes for when you are sleep-deprived. Slow down and watch out that you don't burn yourself on the stove or leave some potentially dangerous thing unattended.

Yes, raising children can be hard on your body. But by exercising preventive measures, you can spare yourself some of the common injuries (and pain) that often occur in motherhood.

11

Frequent Viral Illnesses—Another Occupational Hazard for Moms

At first you hope you're just tired from a busy week. Or maybe you think your scratchy throat is from a change in the weather. Or allergies. But all too soon it becomes apparent—you have another viral illness! Is your new slogan, "I never met a virus I didn't catch"? I expect this is an occupational hazard of motherhood you hadn't expected.

Unfortunately, your precious bundle of joy is a veritable virus magnet during these early years because children have to build their own immunity to all the viruses they come in contact with in the world. This includes hundreds of different viruses that can cause colds, sore throats, bronchitis, conjunctivitis (eye infection), and gastroenteritis (vomiting and diarrhea). The unfair part of this process is that while your child is building immunity to a virus, he or she may show no symptoms but may be contagious enough for *you* to get the virus. When children are coming down with a viral illness, they are contagious before any symptoms appear. That is how these sneaky viruses keep themselves spreading to unsuspecting new victims. Add to this the fact that the average preschooler gets six to ten viral illnesses per year, which means some are getting more than ten each year.[1] It's no wonder you get sick so often (especially in winter). In fact, it's a wonder you are ever well.

There are a few factors that can make you even more vulnerable:

- *Sleep deprivation* weakens the immune system. A single night when you lose three hours of sleep can dramatically reduce your resistance to infection, and the situation will last until you are rested again.
- *Emotional stress and anxiety* make you more susceptible.
- *Pregnant women may be more susceptible* to viruses since their immune systems work differently than usual.
- *At certain times of their menstrual cycle* women can be more susceptible to viral infections.
- *Active allergies of the nasal passages or throat* increase your chances of becoming infected because when these passages are irritated, they are easier to infect.

What Can Be Done to Prevent These Infections?

- *WASH YOUR HANDS after every contact with your child's nasal and mouth secretions.* Cold viruses are spread through nasal and mouth secretions, so washing hands is of utmost importance. Don't leave their used tissues lying around either.
- *Do not touch your eyes, nose, or mouth* after contact with anyone who has a virus. In general, try not to touch your face unless you first wash your hands.
- *Get an annual influenza shot each fall or early winter,* even if you had one the year before, because the influenza virus changes from year to year.
- *Try to get at least seven hours of sleep each night* to keep your immune system strong.

- *A healthy diet and daily multivitamin-mineral supplement* will help your body fight viruses that try to invade. See below for more nutritional supplement help.
- *Exercise* directly increases your immunity. It mobilizes your infection-fighting immune cells as well as relieves stress.

Foiled by Fomites

You will be more successful at preventing viral infections if you watch out for *fomites.* No, these aren't a new strain of termites that feast on foam. Rather they are objects that become contaminated by viruses, which then can transfer viruses to an unsuspecting someone when that person picks up or touches this object. Common fomites include most items used by the sick person, such as used tissues, towels, washcloths, drinking glasses, and teddy bears and other toys that have been handled, sneezed, or slobbered on. Viruses can live on objects for several hours, and they can "infect" the objects just by landing there after being airborne by a sneeze or cough or transmitted by touch.[2] The other surprising thing is how *little* virus you need to come in contact with to become infected—it is truly minuscule amounts![3]

> "How can I avoid getting all the illnesses my child gets?"

Having all this information may not make your cold any better. However, it may help you to realize how difficult it can be to escape a virus that comes home with your child and decides to stay a while. Knowledge is power and, in this case, knowing that fomites are a common carrier can help you avoid obvious objects that could be infected. Be extra careful to wash your hands well after touching such objects.

Good Hand Washing Is Our Best Defense

Let's face it: One of the reasons we get so many viruses from our children is because we are physically involved with them every day—hugging, kissing, snuggling, bathing, playing. Since we are not going to stop doing these things in order to avoid the viruses we catch, our best real physical defense comes down to good hand-washing practices. The biggest key to effective hand washing is *not* that you wash with antibacterial soap. In fact, regular soap may be better since it is not as likely to encourage bacteria to develop resistance to antibacterial measures. The biggest key to effective hand washing is to wash your hands vigorously for at least fifteen seconds with warm water and soap. Here's a tip to help you gauge whether you are washing long enough: Wet your hands, get the soap, then start singing "Happy Birthday" to yourself while you vigorously lather up all parts of your hands. (You may wish to "sing silently" in public, or out loud to teach your kids the same method.) Keep washing until you reach the end of the song, which works out to about fifteen seconds! Then rinse and dry your hands.[4]

Kitchen hand towels as well as drying towels in the bathroom can do more harm than good when it comes to spreading infection, for they easily become fomites. You would be wise to use one paper towel each time you wash instead of the resident towel.

Myths about Viruses

"Stay warm or you'll catch cold." You've probably heard it countless times: "Don't go out without your coat or you'll catch cold." Research done through the National Institute of Allergy and Infectious Diseases tested this common myth. They found that going out in the cold and getting either chilled or overheated does not cause you to "catch cold." There was no relationship between these temperature exposures and the development or worsening of a cold.[5] Instead the connection may be that cold air outside means drier heat indoors, which can dry out your nasal passages, leaving them more susceptible to all the cold viruses that are always looking for "homes" in the winter.

"I just caught this yesterday." Once you are exposed to a virus, the virus percolates in your body for a number of days. This "incubation period" varies from virus to virus, but generally, for the majority of viruses, it is at least two days and up to fourteen days long. In some cases the incubation is as long as several weeks. So if you come down with a cold the very next day after visiting a friend or family member who is fighting a cold, you don't need to regret your visit since not enough time passed for you to have incubated their virus. You picked up *this* one from someone entirely different.

"If he still has a cold, he is still contagious." Once you show symptoms of a cold or other virus, the bad news is that you have already been contagious to others for a day or two. But the good news is that after the symptoms start, with most viral infections you stop being contagious on about the fourth or fifth day of illness.

"We keep passing this cold back and forth." It is a common myth that we pass the same virus back and forth to one another—especially between those who live in our home. This is untrue, because once we have a virus, we build resistance or immunity to it (unless we have a nonfunctional immune system). However, because children (especially preschool children in the winter) get so many viral illnesses and carry even more than they "get," you've likely gotten a brand-new virus if you become ill again right on the heels of another cold, or your initial virus is not yet finished with you. And you're right, *it just isn't fair.*

How to Cope with Frequent Viral Illnesses

So what do you do when you're a mom who needs *your mom* to take care of you? Well, if possible, call your mom for some tender loving care and emotional support, and if she lives nearby, ask her to make some chicken soup and come over. Here are a few ideas to help you cope with the symptoms of yet another viral illness:

Decrease your expectations during these times.

Make homemade chicken soup when you are healthy and freeze portions that you can easily thaw, heat, and eat when you are ill and need them. Whether homemade or canned, this so-called "Jewish penicillin" is more than just a comfort food; well-done studies show there are a number of substances with beneficial medicinal activity in your steaming bowl of soup, especially the broth. A mild anti-inflammatory effect could be one mechanism by which the soup fights against the effects of your cold—so slurp it up![16]

You've heard it before, but remember to drink lots of fluids.

Treat your symptoms of runny nose, mild cough, sore throat, and low-grade fever with over-the-counter medicines as needed to help you be more comfortable. Use acetaminophen for aches and fever, over-the-counter cold medicines for day relief, and consider liquid Nyquil for nighttime relief because it may help you sleep.

Oral antibiotics will not *help unless a complication seems to have occurred,* such as nasal discharge that is now cloudy green, feeling much sicker instead of better after four or five days of illness, having a new higher fever after several days of illness, or developing a severe cough.

Puffs Plus tissues or Kleenex Ultra are worth the extra cost when you have a cold because they pamper your tender, sore nose.

Sleep as much as possible because it helps your body conquer the virus more quickly.

Rest especially in the first twenty-four to forty-eight hours. Sometimes you can decrease the overall severity of the illness with rest at the beginning.

If there is someone who can help with the children and your duties, enlist their aid so you can rest.

Nutritional Supplements May Help

Is there an herbal or natural cure for colds? So far research has not confirmed that a magical substance exists to prevent our viral misery. But we do know that it is easier to catch viruses and harder to get rid of them if our diets are deficient in nutrients. So once again, I strongly recommend that you take a daily multivitamin and mineral supplement in addition to making certain you eat at least five servings of fruits and vegetables each day.

What about vitamin C? Several large-scale controlled studies have been done in both adults and children, but as of now none has confirmed the belief that taking large doses of vitamin C will prevent colds. However, studies suggest vitamin C may decrease the severity of symptoms and shorten the course of the illness.[7]

There are a few other commonly used herbal, vitamin, and mineral remedies that may or may not help you feel better:

Echinacea. This member of the daisy family is an herbal supplement that can be helpful as an immune system booster. For some people, echinacea appears to at least shorten the course of an illness as well as decrease the symptoms of a cold (up to 50 to 60 percent in one study).[8] It may work better once you get a cold than as a cold prevention herb. Do not take it for more than eight to ten weeks straight or it may decrease your immune function rather than strengthen it. Please note: Pregnant or nursing women should not take echinacea.

Goldenseal. This member of the buttercup family is commonly combined with echinacea and promoted as a cold and flu remedy. There are no good studies on goldenseal that confirm it is effective against colds. If you are going to take echinacea, I recommend leaving the goldenseal behind in the buttercup patch.

Astragalus. This Chinese root has been used for centuries in Chinese medicine, which claims it stimulates the immune system in patients with infections.[9] Studies on its ability to boost the immune system have been sparse but promising. In one clinical trial in the U.S., the root was shown to increase the number of infection-fighting white blood cells (T cells) in some patients with cancer.[10] If you wish to try astragalus, one good way is in a combination formula with echinacea.

Airborne Effervescent Dietary Supplement. Airborne contains seven Chinese herbs (including echinacea and ginger) and some vitamins, minerals, and amino acids (the building blocks of protein) in a tablet. Drop this tasty orange-flavored fizzy tablet into a glass of water and drink it. This over-the-counter supplement may reduce the symptoms of newly developed upper respiratory infection—and they have clinical research to support that claim. The GNG Pharmaceutical company conducted a double-blind, placebo controlled, multi-center, randomized clinical trial using Airborne. In other words, the most reliable type of clinical research was completed. They studied adults above the age of eighteen who just developed cold symptoms within the previous twenty-four hours. The study found that 79 percent of the Airborne users had at least a partial decrease in symptoms, while only 23 percent of the placebo users reported a benefit. Those studied reported no adverse effects of any kind with either Airborne or the placebo.[11] Does this mean Airborne will work for you? It's impossible to say, but the results of this first clinical study are encouraging. It is also comforting that there were no adverse effects associated with the product; however, women who are pregnant or breastfeeding should not take Airborne.

Zinc lozenges. Recent studies with the mineral zinc in lozenge form show there was some relief of cold symptoms (especially runny nose and cough) and shortening of the course of the illness.[12] The study compared adult cold sufferers who took higher dose zinc lozenges (13 to 23 mg of zinc) several times a day with cold sufferers who took a placebo. But other studies have not confirmed benefits when lower dose lozenges were used (5 mg or less).[13] *Note that zinc lozenges should never be given to children.*

Sambucol (black elderberry extract). This "elderberry syrup" called Sambucol is not what you pour on your pancakes, but it could help you fight influenza. In a double-blind, placebo-controlled, randomized study, Sambucol reduced the duration of influenza symptoms to three to four days (compared to six days for those not on Sambucol). In addition, the blood antibody levels measured after the infection were higher in the group that took the Sambucol, suggesting that there was a stronger immune response.[14] Another recent study showed that Sambucol stimulated the immune response in healthy volunteers.[15] More studies are needed to confirm Sambucol's effectiveness, but so far results sound promising and tasty.

The Long-Range Forecast

Viral infections are one of those rare things a mother wishes her child wouldn't share with her. But the fact remains that getting those virus infections is an occupational hazard of being a loving and caring mom. The good news is that children don't remain the virus magnets they once were; they grow past that stage as they age beyond their preschool years. So take heart, because the long-range forecast is for fewer blustery colds and runny noses in the seasons ahead.

12

The Benefits of Wise Lifestyle Choices

> The acts of the sinful nature are obvious: sexual immorality, impurity and debauchery; idolatry and witchcraft; hatred, discord, jealousy, fits of rage, selfish ambition, dissensions, factions and envy; drunkenness, orgies, and the like.
>
> Galatians 5:19–21

Throughout your time here at the MOPS Spa we have covered many wise choices that go a long way toward helping you and your family maintain good health. However, we still need to address one group of sensitive topics. Each one can bring serious harm to your health when the wrong choice is made. These issues are smoking, excessive alcohol intake, drug abuse, overspending, overeating, and extramarital affairs. With most of these issues, you already know the "right thing to do," even though making the right choice may be difficult because it means you have to give up something that has an unhealthy hold on you. It's time to break down the barriers and openly discuss these issues. I hope this will help you summon the courage to do what you need to do to break free from any of these that affect your life.

Breaking Free from Unhealthy Reactions to Stress

Each of us is human. Period. We find ourselves with vices and habits that we know are not good for us, but still we persist with them. This is not a chapter to condemn you for your vices. Rather it is meant to inform, encourage, and ultimately help you break the hold these vices have on you and your health. As the apostle Paul reminds us, "It is for freedom that Christ has set us free. Stand firm, then, and do not let yourselves be burdened again by a yoke of slavery" (Galatians 5:1).

> *"I do not understand what I do. For what I want to do I do not do, but what I hate I do. . . . What a wretched man I am! Who will rescue me from this body of death? Thanks be to God—through Jesus Christ our Lord!"*
>
> *—Romans 7:15, 24–25*

What do all of these issues have in common? Each can begin out of an attempt to escape the effects of stress or to deal with feelings of stress. But the irony is that in the long run, each of these coping mechanisms causes more stress and pain than it ever relieved. Underlying these lifestyle choices can be anger, stress, anxiety, fear, a very painful memory you are trying to flee, broken dreams, or unmet expectations. Any of these may have started the coping mechanism, but soon the habit takes on a life and a hold all its own. Your body becomes addicted to the nicotine coursing through your bloodstream, alcohol asks for more and more, and drugs like the painkiller Vicodin can quickly cause dependence.

Extramarital Affairs: The Tender Trap

Illicit sexual behavior also is very "addictive." Many women become addicted to the excitement of "forbidden fruit," a new romance. The chemicals and hormones released in the bloodstream during an affair are like a drug. Even though women may feel guilty, they "crave" more of this "drug" once the most recent meeting is over, which just perpetuates the vicious cycle of seeking the next rendezvous.

Extramarital affairs are more common than you may think among both Christians and non-Christians. According to Maggie Scarf, author of *Intimate Partners,* "Most experts consider the 'educated guess' at the present time . . . [is] 45–55 percent of wives [are] extra-maritally involved by age 40."[1] Affairs are attractive because they offer dramatic distraction from all that is bothering you—that is, for the moment. But then you end up much more stressed as guilt, worry about being caught, and conflict with all your values erupt from your conscience. Plus you realize you may be at risk for pregnancy and sexually transmitted diseases.

If this coping choice has directly touched your life, there is hope. You can break free from this destructive trap. You can be healed from the destructive effects on your faith, your marriage, and your self-esteem, but usually that means you need the help of a counselor who will help you realize why this started in the first place and then will hold you accountable as you break your addiction to the affair.

Addictions Are "Normal"

With all this talk about "addiction," what would you say if I told you it is normal to have addictions? Nancy Deason, MFCC, a Christian counselor who treats many Christian women with addictions, explains why this is so:

> Everyone has addictions. The issue is whether they are healthy addictions or unhealthy addictions. The power of any addiction is that it can change how we feel. When we feel an unpleasant feeling that we don't want to feel, we unconsciously

are driven to escape that feeling by looking for a different feeling. . . . And we are all going to be dependent on anything that can reduce our anxiety; . . . fear is at the heart of addictions. One mark of a high functioning life is whether a person has the ability to self-soothe in a healthy way. These would be "smart addictions" as they can be done without cost, in daytime or evenings, and not create any secondary problems. Some examples would be needlepoint, reading, photography, genealogy, memory albums, art, journaling, etc. Addictions can keep us in chains of despair while we lose control of our lives . . . or they can be rewarding to us and at the same time be healthy modeling to our families.

What Can Motivate Us Enough to Break Free?

When we have an addiction that is an unhealthy habit, probably the most potent vehicle for personal change is when you know it adversely affects your children. The second would be when you know you have a health problem that can turn fatal if you continue the habit. Many smokers have finally broken their addictions to cigarettes because of these two factors.

The Smoke Trap

Of all these issues, smoking probably is the most potentially harmful to you and your children. It not only affects your children indirectly by putting their mother at risk for lung cancer and increasing your risk of heart attack and stroke, but it directly harms them through secondhand smoke. Children are at risk for conditions such as asthma, frequent bronchitis, lung cancer, heart disease, and stroke, even if they personally never take a puff.[2] In the Nurses' Health Study, those who were nonsmokers but exposed to secondhand smoke regularly in either home or office settings had a 91 percent increased risk of heart attack, compared to those not exposed to secondhand smoke![3]

Many smokers truly do not understand how much smoke they expose their children to. "I always smoke outside," and "I always smoke with the car window down," and finally, "I never smoke in the car when the kids are inside," are the responses I have heard from countless, well-meaning moms and dads who have not yet broken their tobacco addiction. But the problem is, every one of those situations is still putting your children at great risk. Even if you always smoke outside, smoke remains on your clothes and in your lungs, so it is breathed right into your child's face when you talk, cuddle, and kiss your child. If you ever smoke in a car, the toxic fumes penetrate the upholstery and carpet and leech out into the air when your children ride in that vehicle.

It's Time to Kick the Habit

I know this is difficult to hear if you are a mom who smokes. Though you would never want to hurt your children, this is one habit that does. It is time to take action and quit! For those of you who have attempted to quit but were unsuccessful in the past, research confirms that it is both psychologically and biochemically more difficult for women to quit than it is for men.[4] Only 4 percent of those who try to quit smoking "cold turkey" without any outside help are still nonsmokers after a year, so that means you need to take advantage of all the help you can find to beat the odds. The Breath of Fresh Air website at www.4woman.gov/QuitSmoking is a great place to start your search for information about all the helps available to you. When you quit smoking you are breaking two addictions: your body's biochemical dependence on nicotine and your psychological attachment to cigarettes. Smoking is something you associate doing with many daily activities such as lighting up right after dinner or while talking on the phone. That means you need to treat both addictions to kick the habit. Talk with your doctor about products such as the nicotine patch, Nicorette gum, and even Zyban, an oral medication that can help. Joining a support group is usually a key to success. *You can do it*—but you probably need help to succeed.

Series of Health Benefits When You Quit Smoking

The minute you quit smoking, your body starts to recover. After . . .

20 minutes: Blood pressure and heart rate become nearly normal

2 hours: Nicotine starts to leave your system

8 hours: Oxygen and carbon dioxide levels in blood normalize

12 hours: Carbon monoxide has left your system

1 day: Your risk of heart attack starts to decrease

1 week: Sense of smell and taste return, and nicotine is out of your system

2 weeks: Circulation becomes better and breathing improves

1–2 months: Mucus starts to clear out of lungs, coughing decreases, and energy increases

1 year: Your risk of heart disease is now less than half of what it was a year ago!

5 years: Your risk of cancer of lung, mouth, and throat is half of a pack-a-day smoker's

10 years: Your risk of dying of lung cancer is now similar to a nonsmoker's[5]

Let's Get You Free!

My best advice when you are caught in the trap of any habit is to seek professional help to break free. Admitting you need help is not a sign of weakness but a sign that you are smart enough to recognize that there is a serious hold on the life God gave you. By admitting there is a problem, you demonstrate that you honor him and your family and yourself enough to get the help you need, knowing you can't break free alone. Once you have taken the steps necessary and made the wise choice, you will reap the benefits of an abundant life without this hold.

Unfortunately, there usually is shame involved with these habits, which makes you even more diligent about not wanting to tell anyone about the more secretive ones. Shame is like super-vitamins to this vicious cycle. Because you are ashamed, you feel more anxious and depressed; because you are more anxious and depressed, you seek the comfort of your habit to make you feel better—which makes you feel ashamed. Enough already! Let's get you free. Who can you call today to help you get the help you need? A Christian counselor? Your physician? A smoking cessation support group? Take that first step towards freedom and the rest will follow, with God as your partner every step of the way.

Special Bonus Section: Wisely Choose Your Household Cleaning Supplies

"Cleanliness is next to godliness," right? But cleaning with many common household cleaners can be hazardous to your health and the health of your loved ones. It is time to reevaluate what products you are using to clean your home and see if there are wiser choices to be made.

What's the big deal? More and more research confirms that the air pollution inside our homes is far worse than the air outside our homes. In fact, over the last decade, the U.S. Environmental Protection Agency has consistently ranked indoor air pollution among the top five risks to public health.[6] Many usual cleaners—such as chlorine containing Clorox, ammonia-containing cleaners, caustic cleaners like Tilex, and phosphate-containing detergents and dishwasher soaps all emit potentially harmful gases into the air. These gases are called VOCs (Volatile Organic Compounds). One little-known fact is that even when you are not actively using toxic cleaners, they continue to send fumes into the air from under the sink or wherever you store them. It's called "out gassing."[7] This means that you and your family are continually exposed to the health-damaging effects of these cleaners. Even more dangerous is if you combine some of these cleaners (like Clorox and ammonia), for this creates very toxic gases that are very hazardous to your health, even fatal.

Ironically, if you currently use these products, it probably is because you are trying to kill the household germs that may be harmful to your children. But the cure may be more harmful than the germs. Exposure to these substances often causes more than just temporary irritation to your breathing passages and eyes. Studies show severe irritation to breathing passageways and even lung damage following exposure to chlorine gas–containing cleaners (like Clorox). Scientists that study the effects of toxic gases on humans confirm that using certain home cleaners can be as dangerous to your health as being near a hazardous chemical spill. "Symptoms and signs following inhalation of mixtures of chlorine-containing cleaners in the home are similar to those after occupational exposures and environmental releases.... Controlled human exposure data suggest that some subjects (like children) may be more responsive to the effects of chlorine and may be at greater risk of adverse outcome after chlorine inhalation."[8] Studies also link use of these home cleaners with bronchitis and the increased development of asthma in many people.[9] There also is a sobering fifteen-year study done in Oregon, which found that those women who worked at home had a 54 percent higher death rate from cancer than women who worked at jobs away from home.[10] The study suggested that the continuous exposure to household cleaners might be the main reason for this difference.

It is a safe assumption that if you feel like you need a gas mask in order to clean your shower, then you probably are using a cleaner that could damage your health. Instead, consider buying or making nontoxic and natural cleaners to protect your entire family. When shopping for cleaners, check the labels for caustic agents such as those listed above. Some examples of effective, nontoxic cleaning products include the Ecosense cleaning line from Melaleuca, the Wellness Company,[11] the Miracle Clean product line by Joy Mangano,[12] and the widely available product that has been around for twenty-five years, Simple Green.[13] An excellent resource for recipes to make your own cleaners from common products such as baking soda and vinegar is the website of the new Christian ministry Healthy Families, Healthy Environment, at www.healthy familiesnow.org.

If you decide to keep the cleaners you have, read the label carefully and follow all safety guidelines, such as using gloves and allowing excellent ventilation during and after use. Also, when you are cleaning, please keep your children away from the area, since their little bodies are much more susceptible to all the damaging effects.[14]

Part Three

Understanding the Complexities of Female Chemistry

13

Libido, Libido . . . Where's My Libido?

Help! My Sex Drive Drove Away!

It's very distressing to realize you suddenly have no desire for sex—or at most very little desire. This is a common concern for moms, especially in the first months after delivery. Many say jokingly that having a young child is one of the most reliable methods of birth control, because libido (or desire for sex) seems to vanish. In other words, the exhaustion, lack of sleep, and life-altering impact that follow having children often leave parents with little interest in or energy for their sex life; the situation can even discourage them from wanting to add any more little ones to their flock.

> *"How can I regain my 'libido' or desire for sex?"*

However, sex and intimate time with your mate is very important during this time. You need the energizing release that lovemaking brings. And at a time when you are both so focused on your children, you need to consciously decide to focus on each other.

Loss of libido is a complicated issue because it can be caused by many different physical, emotional, and social factors. An expert who can help sort out the complexities of female chemistry is Dr. Colleen McNally, who not only has a busy private practice in ob-gyn but also is chairman of the Bioethics Department for San Diego Sharp Hospitals and vice-chief of the Department of Obstetrics and Gynecology at Sharp Hospital. Dr. McNally is a mother of three: Mike, age twelve; Connor, ten; and Catherine, eight. Yes, she's even a tried-and-true soccer mom. As both a doctor and a mother, she too remembers those low libido days when her children were very young. "It is such an overwhelming time, and you are so exhausted. After working all day and caring for the kids, the last thing I wanted was someone to touch me. I should stress that loss of libido is very, very normal. If you're not sleeping, you're stressed, and you're not exercising, your libido will not be there."

There are reasons for your decreased libido.

- *Immediate postpartum.* You have at least a six-week waiting period following delivery for one reason. This is a time for recovery. Some women have no libido because they worry there may be pain with intercourse after having a child, especially if an episiotomy was necessary.
- *Hormones.* The many fluctuations of hormone levels following birth can cause your desire to fizzle temporarily.
- *Certain medications.* Certain antidepressants and blood pressure medications (beta-blockers) can decrease libido.
- *The changes in your body from pregnancy.* This can include changes in your breast size or how they now sag, increased weight where there wasn't extra before, or a lesser level of fitness if not able to exercise regularly. All of these can understandably make moms feel less desirable.
- *Exhaustion and sleep deprivation.* These two are inevitable when you're caring for your child day and night.
- *The business of mothering.* It is hard to feel sexy when you are consumed by the tasks at hand: shampooing heads,

cleaning up the "Picasso masterpiece" that your two-year-old just created with his lunch on the drop cloth under his chair, and enduring your willful four-year-old's tantrums that you find are so much worse than those he had in the so-called "terrible twos."

- *A change of focus.* The radical change in your perspective, from being a wife in love with only your husband to being a mother focused and unbelievably in love with your child, changes how you approach physical intimacy.

Getting It Back

Make Your Communication Sizzle

We all know communication with our spouse is key if we want to have a great marriage and sex life. But how does this work once you become parents? No longer do you have the luxury of those leisurely talks over dinner, without interruptions, just the two of you. Without setting aside time regularly to talk through the issues in your marriage and family life, those issues don't get resolved. You are more likely to get burned by "stewing" problems that suddenly boil over and create a big mess. Plus, now that you have children, there is even more you need to talk about yet less time to do it. Very often the cozy talks about your relationship get "shoved to the back burner" or end up "off the stove" entirely. It's not realistic to expect that you will be "hot" for each other when you each have resentments simmering on a back burner. First, "heat up" over some tasty conversation. Here are some truths and tips for cooking up gourmet communication:

If you are angry with your husband and do not discuss it or resolve it, your feelings will morph into resentment (which is like that baked-on stuff on the bottom of a pan—it's very hard to get rid of).

Do you have differing expectations about what amount of the family workload each of you should shoulder? Dr. McNally recommends you "tell your husband if he wants a more active sex life right now, he's got to help out more." Be specific about what you expect and what you can and cannot do. Then find a compromise that you both can live with. One effective way to do this is to sit down together and make a list of all the household duties and childcare responsibilities, then write in the name of who is responsible for what. Having it on paper gives both of you a clear place to start.

Try at least once a month—preferably once a week—to sit down with both of your calendars and discuss what events, commitments, and scheduled items are ahead. Also reevaluate whether you are both "happy enough" with your division of family work. If not, keep trying to find the right balance.

Talk about how parenthood has changed your sex life. Just discussing this issue openly can open up both of you to new possibilities. Try to find the humor hidden in this challenge. By not taking it so seriously you can reopen the door to playing and loving together. You will also not be isolated with thoughts such as, "He doesn't want me anymore," or "I don't feel attractive enough to make love," or even, "What is wrong with me—I have no sex drive!"

Remember, you *do* still have a sex drive. It's just squashed right now by the enormous task of parenthood itself and all that comes along with it physically, emotionally, and mentally.

Get Physical So You'll Want to Get Physical

One of the many marvelous benefits of exercise is that it may improve your ability to be sexually aroused. That benefit alone could mean it's worth running around the block a few extra times.

There also is a specific exercise, called the Kegel exercise, that may boost your libido, sexual function, and urination control. Essentially this exercise works the muscle in the area of your urethra (where urine comes out) and vaginal opening, called the pubococcygeus, or PC muscle, in the area called the pelvic floor. The Kegel exercise strengthens the pelvic floor and may directly increase your libido and improve vaginal lubrication and tightness, make it easier for you to reach orgasm, and stop stress incontinence (when urine leaks out with laughing, sneezing, and exercising, which many women experience after childbirth).

To benefit from Kegel, it's important to do the Kegel exercise properly. Make sure you are working the right muscle. You can find it by trying to stop the flow of urine when you are voiding. Another way to confirm it is to place your finger in your vaginal opening and then squeeze that muscle. If you feel pressure around your finger, you have found the right muscle. Once you've found the right muscle, contract it for a count of four, then relax for a count of four.

One way to think of it is to imagine that the pelvic floor is an elevator. On contraction the elevator goes up, and with relaxation the elevator comes down. Finally, for best results, this exercise should be done for five minutes two times each day.[1]

Add "Date Night" to Your Vocabulary

If you haven't already done so, you need to add this new term to your vocabulary: *Date Night.* It is one of the easiest things to forget about in the midst of the hustle and bustle of family life, but also one of the best ways to improve your marriage. I cannot emphasize enough how crucial it is that you do this. Dates allow you to change your focus from kid-vision to spouse-vision—even if only for a few hours. To make it happen, swap babysitting with another mom so that both your families can benefit from dates. You need not do anything expensive on your dates. Even spending the time taking a drive together, watching a sunset, or having an uninterrupted cup of coffee at a restaurant will do.

The key to positive results from a date night is to try to rediscover why you fell in love with this man. Flirt with him rather than talking about the need for a termite inspection. Focus on your husband, not on what might be happening at home.

Without this type of focus, your marriage could be at risk. If you don't remember why you love your spouse, it can eat away the foundation of your marriage, weakening the bonds you share as a couple. Scenarios of resentment, attraction to others outside of your marriage, and other dangers can all be avoided if you take care of this crucial relationship. Your marriage is the most important relationship in your family. If you do not feed it and strengthen it, the foundation may crumble beneath you.

Especially helpful to marriages and your sex life are overnight get-away dates. Even if much of the time you find yourselves thinking about and talking about the kids, getting away from the house with just the two of you can do amazing things for your passion. Again, this need not be expensive. In fact, a night at Motel 6 with "the magic fingers" massager attached to the bed is quite low in cost yet high in fun. God gave you the gift of sex to enjoy with your husband, so let yourself enjoy each other. Be sure to wear something that helps you feel sexy and desirable.

Just Show Up

Even when you feel exhausted and aren't particularly interested in a passionate romp, often if you will just "show up" and join in the love-making with your husband, the feelings and arousal will catch up with you. And that sexual release will likely give you more energy and relieve stress (in addition to adding a rosy bloom to your face).

Schedule Sex on Your Calendar

I realize it doesn't sound very romantic to schedule sex on the calendar, but this fact remains: When you have more sex, you want sex more. But sex is not likely to happen unless you make a clear choice to have it. Take out your calendar and together decide which night(s) and what time you are going to make love. Another advantage to this approach is you can both anticipate it, which can make your sexual pleasure even greater.

Shoot for the Moon!

I have my husband's permission to tell you about the best Christmas present he thinks I've ever given to him. I was reading a women's magazine at the hair salon a few years ago when I came across an article that suggested married couples with kids should plan to have sex every night. As I read on, the author (herself a mother of two) told of how this plan revolutionized her and her husband's sex life. By planning to make love every night, it meant that quickies were okay, and every time did not have to be the end-all of lovemaking episodes. So I took the challenge and wrote up a certificate for my husband, offering him nightly romps from Christmas Eve onward. I don't think I've ever seen him smile so much! I was still skeptical about whether this was feasible—and if I could survive such a pace, but this plan turned out so much better than I anticipated. The every-night aspect did not continue more than a week or so, but I must say that since we both had the expectation that we would be together each night, it strangely took pressure *off* of our sex life. It brought us closer in all respects because we took on this challenge. So now you know the perfect Christmas present for your hubby! But why wait for Christmas?

Blocking the Pass?

If you still lack the desire to make love, ask yourself if you are blocking advances from your mate. If so, explore what the reasons are: Is it because you think the only time he touches you is when he wants sex (anger), or because you are not sure about your own performance ("I haven't done it for so long I'm not sure I know how!"), or perhaps for another reason altogether? Again, it helps tremendously to talk with your husband about the reasons you have for blocking him (and vice versa).

Sex therapists routinely advise couples to stop all intercourse for a period of time (usually up to a few weeks) and instead spend time together cuddling, kissing, touching, and talking. Intercourse is not allowed. This takes the pressure off, allowing you to rekindle the desire you have for one another and encouraging you to enjoy each other's touch again. And usually, before you know it, *you* will be breaking the "no intercourse" rule and asking him to make love!

WANTED: A Woman's Lost Libido

If you have done what you can do and your libido is a still a fugitive, it is time to consult your ob-gyn doctor to rule out any major hormonal or physical reasons for this change. If it is any consolation, remember that a loss of libido is very common among mothers. Think about it this way—you *will* likely find your sex drive again because we know it exists or you and your husband would not be parents in the first place!

14

Safe Birth Control

We are fortunate to have many different types of safe birth control available. But since there is such great variety, choosing can be confusing. What is right for this season of your marriage and mothering may be quite different than what is best for you later on. In addition, the physical effects of certain methods can make them a healthy choice for some women and not healthy for others.

You can simplify the complex decision of which one is safest and healthiest for you if you consider the different methods available in light of this series of questions:

> *"What are the safest, healthiest forms of birth control?"*

How crucial is it that I not get pregnant? If it is vitally important to you that you not get pregnant, then it is best to choose a method with a very low failure rate, such as oral contraceptives or Depo-Provera.

What will my husband and I use every time? It doesn't matter how effective a method is supposed to be if you will not use it every time. So be as honest as possible with yourself. Will you remember to take a birth control pill every day? Are you willing to interrupt your lovemaking to insert foam or for your husband to don a condom? Will you plan ahead to insert a diaphragm before lovemaking? Or would you rather have a Depo-Provera shot that lasts for three months? Only you and your husband know the answers.

Are there side effects with this method that I cannot tolerate? This issue is very personal and very important, so pay attention. Since every woman's body is unique, you may experience side effects with some forms of birth control that are different than those of other women. For instance, some women have pain with the IUD, some have very strong mood swings on Depo-Provera, and others have weight gain and moodiness on oral contraceptives. Yet there are also women who use each of these methods without suffering any side effects. I know it can be frustrating to try a method and find it's not right for you, but work with your doctor to hone in on which is the best fit with your personal body chemistry.

Do I want temporary or permanent birth control? Most forms of birth control are temporary, but there also are more permanent options. For women, there is tubal ligation ("getting your tubes tied"), and for men, the vasectomy (getting his "tubes" tied); both are considered minor surgical procedures, but a tubal ligation is a much more complicated surgery than a vasectomy. There are many other issues you must think through if permanent birth control seems right for you. How old are you now? Some doctors strongly discourage permanent measures if you are still very young. Is there *any* chance that you might wish to get pregnant in the future? What if your child died? Would you then consider getting pregnant again? These are tough questions to face, but they are important to ask before you make this decision.

Is there a birth control method that could improve our sex life? Think about how your current birth control method impacts your actual lovemaking. If you are using a barrier method like condom, foam, or diaphragm, is the insertion or interruption negatively affecting your enjoyment of sex? Are you still afraid you will get pregnant with your current method? The right birth control method can increase your libido and enjoyment of sex, especially if other methods are interfering directly or giving you concern that pregnancy could happen.

How does the birth control method work to prevent pregnancy? This question is especially important if you are concerned whether a fertilized egg could be involved in the method you are considering. It is still a difficult question to answer for some methods of birth control. Obviously condoms work by keeping the sperm from getting to the egg. Foam works by killing the sperm before they can make the journey. Some controversy still exists about whether IUDs and some of the hormonal contraceptives work in part by not allowing a fertilized egg to implant in the endometrium—in other words, does the body sometimes "abort" a fertilized egg when these methods are used?

Most experts believe that oral contraceptives (combination pills) work most of the time by suppressing ovulation, so there is no egg to worry about. If a woman does ovulate while on the combination pill, there is still another deterrent, for this pill makes the cervical mucus thick and hostile toward sperm, so the sperm do not get past this "guard" and can't move on toward the egg. Despite these main ways that the combination pill prevents pregnancy, experts know that at times fertilization of eggs still occurs. When it does occur, the combo pill may work by preventing implantation. I wish I could tell you how often this occurs, but the medical science jury is still out, and there is no consensus about if or when this happens. (See the appendix: CMDA Statement on Hormonal Contraception and Abortion for discussion by experts from the Christian Medical & Dental Associations.)

The mini-pill (progesterone only) works differently than the combination pill. Since it has no estrogen, its main action is not to stop ovulation. However, it too makes the cervical mucus thick, hostile, and hard for sperm to pass through. But in the case of the mini-pill, there is a much greater concern that the other mini-pill action—keeping the uterine lining from thickening—may prevent a fertilized egg that could potentially come to the uterus from being able to implant. According to Gene Rudd, M.D., an obstetrician-gynecologist and the associate executive director of the Christian Medical & Dental Associations, "While [progesterone-only products] may inhibit ovulation, by design they must work at least part of the time after fertilization."[1] Again, it is difficult to know how often this occurs. (See the appendix for the CMDA statement on hormonal contraception and abortion.)

The same concern also exists for IUD products. According to Dr. Rudd, "As for IUDs, while the copper and progesterone IUDs have decreased the occurrence of post-fertilization effects, they remain a significant mechanism of action."[2] So, although the main action of IUDs is believed to prevent pregnancy by immobilizing sperm on their way to the egg, there still is the possibility that fertilized eggs are being turned away from implantation.

The Whole Scoop on Different Methods of Birth Control

This section is a resource to provide you with information on the many forms of birth control available. We will spotlight each type of method, how it works, its effectiveness, disadvantages, safety issues, cost approximations, and other important tidbits of information drawn from a number of sources.[3] For additional information I highly recommend the resource book *1001 Health-Care Questions Women Ask* by obstetrician-gynecologist Dr. Joe S. McIlhaney Jr., and Susan Nethery.[4]

Hormonal Types

This category includes hormones in pill form, injectable form, and forms you place on or inside your body.

Combination Oral Contraceptives ($25/month)

What is it? Known by most as "the pill," or combined pill, it is a daily pill that contains both synthetic estrogen and progesterone hormones that are taken every day for twenty-one days, then without hormones for seven days (to have a period). Those with 20 to 35 micrograms estrogen and low dose progesterone usually work well for most women. Higher dose forms are also available.

How does it work? By suppressing the ovaries from ovulating. It also makes the cervical mucus thick and hostile toward sperm, not allowing the sperm to get through. It may also work by preventing fertilized eggs from implanting in the uterus.

Advantages: Dr. McNally confirms that studies show "it greatly reduces your lifetime risk (by 70 percent) for ovarian cancer if you have taken the pill seven years or longer. It decreases the risk of benign ovarian cysts, ruptured ovarian cysts, and endometriosis. Some studies show that women on the pill in their forties prior to menopause enter menopause with a higher bone density than those women not on the pill. Fertility usually returns the month after you stop taking the pills."

Disadvantages: You must remember to take them every day or the method is not effective. You can have weight gain, mood swings, a bloated feeling, nausea, and spotting between periods.

> "How long is it safe for me to be on the pill? All the way to menopause?"

Effectiveness: Nearly 100 percent if used correctly; actual about 97 percent.

Safety issues: Estrogen can increase the risk of blood clots, cardiovascular disease, high blood pressure, heart attacks, and stroke, and increase the chance of gallstones.

According to Dr. Colleen McNally, the latest research confirms that "birth control pills are very safe to take all the way to menopause *unless* you are over the age of thirty-five and also smoke. Be careful if you have a history of hypertension. There is also evidence that if you have a history of migraines with aura that you have increased risk of stroke, even though the risk of stroke while you are on the pill is very, very low. Plus the dosages on the pill are so much lower than they were fifteen years ago."

Beware of the drug interactions that can happen with the pill and other drugs like antibiotics (tetracycline, ampicillin) and anticonvulsants (phenobarbital, Tegretol, phenytoin). The other drug can decrease the effectiveness of the pill, and you could become pregnant. Ask your doctor if there could be a possible interaction with any other medications you take. Your doctor may prescribe a higher dose birth control pill or suggest you use an additional form of birth control.

Mini-Pill ($25/month)

What is it? Progesterone-only hormone pill.

How does it work? Makes cervical mucus thick and hostile to sperm so they cannot reach egg. May decrease uterine lining, which affects whether fertilized egg can implant.

Advantages: Great for breastfeeding moms.

Disadvantages: Must be taken at the same time every day. If late taking the pill, a backup birth control must be used for forty-eight hours. Not quite as effective as combination pill. May cause some irregular bleeding. Can have breast tenderness, moodiness, and weight gain.

Effectiveness: 95 percent.

Safety issues: Minimal concerns.

Depo-Provera Shot ($40 to $70/3 months)

What is it? An injection of 150 mg of long-acting progesterone. It is projected to keep a woman from getting pregnant for three months, though in some cases the effect lasts longer.

How does it work? Suppresses ovulation.

Advantages: Very effective birth control for three months without any daily pill to remember.

Disadvantages: Women may have irregular bleeding throughout the entire three months, weight gain, breast tenderness, and headaches. Once the injection is in, it cannot be removed, so the patient may have to go through three months of side effects. Periods may not resume right after the three-month mark—can take a year in some cases.

Effectiveness: Nearly 100 percent; as effective as tubal ligation, but this method is reversible.

Safety issues: Minimal concerns.

Lunelle Injection ($30 to $35/month)

What is it? Injectable form of progesterone and estrogen taken once a month.

How does it work? Similar to the combined pill.

Advantages: Not having to remember to take daily birth control pills.

Disadvantages: You have to remember when to go in for next injection.

Effectiveness: 94 to 99 percent.

Safety issues: Similar to combined pill.

Vaginal Contraceptive Ring ($25 to $35/month)

What is it? A 2.5 cm ring containing estrogen and progesterone that women insert high in the vagina and leave in for three weeks. The hormones are released slowly and absorbed for three weeks. Then the ring is removed for one week. The woman gets her menstrual period, and then a new ring needs to be inserted.

How does it work? Similar to combined pill.

Advantages: Not having to remember to take daily birth control pills.

Disadvantages: Must remember when to change ring; vaginal discharge/irritation for some.

Effectiveness: 94 to 99 percent.

Safety issues: Similar to combined pill.

Pill Patch ($30 to $35/month)

What is it? Skin patch worn for three weeks on the lower abdomen, buttocks, or upper body that releases the hormones progesterone and estrogen into the bloodstream. The patch is removed for one week to have a menstrual period. New patch is then attached.

How does it work? Similar to combined pill.

Advantages: Not having to remember to take daily birth control pills.

Disadvantages: Have to remember when to change patch *and* make sure patch is attached securely.

Effectiveness: 94 to 99 percent. Less effective if woman weighs over 198 pounds.

Safety issues: Similar to combined pill.

IUDs: Intrauterine Devices

There are three types of IUDs available:

- *Paraguard* (can be left in for ten years)—contains copper; can cause heavier periods ($300 to $500/10 years)
- *Progestersert* (must be changed every year)—contains progesterone hormone ($400/year)
- *Mirena* (can be in for five years)—contains progesterone; may cause decreased bleeding from periods ($400/5 years)

What is it? A T-shaped device that is inserted into the uterus by a doctor. It prevents pregnancy anywhere from one to twelve years, depending on the type used.

How does it work? It immobilizes sperm so they cannot penetrate the egg. May also work to prevent implantation of fertilized egg in uterus.

Advantages: Very effective birth control without any daily pills to take or barrier methods to remember to use.

Disadvantages: Possible pelvic infection in first three months of use. Cramping, bleeding, and pelvic pain can all be side effects.

Effectiveness: 97 percent.

Safety issues: According to Dr. Colleen McNally, "IUDs got a bad reputation with the Dalkon shield [type] in the '70s because it had a string that allowed bacteria to cling to it and climb up the string and cause infection. The new IUDs have string that the bacteria cannot cling to, so the incidence of pelvic inflammatory disease is very low. There is a slight increase in pelvic infections the first three months after it has been inserted, but for women who are in monogamous relationships, the risk of developing pelvic infections is very low. A low risk of uterus perforation does exist."

Barrier Methods

The biggest drawback to barrier methods in general is that you must remember to use them every time you make love. Depending on which method you choose, some require insertion or application just before intercourse.

Condom with Spermicidal Foam (condoms $0.50 to $3/use), (spermicide $0.50 to $3/use)

- *Latex or polyurethane* (if allergic to latex). Protects against sexually transmitted diseases (STDs).
- *Lambskin or natural.* Feel more natural, but they do not protect against STDs.
- *Reality female condoms.* These are only 75 percent effective against pregnancy when used alone, but do protect against STDs.

What is it? Also known as a "rubber," a condom is a tubelike sheath that is sealed at one end; it slips onto the man's penis when erect and catches semen during intercourse.

How does it work? Prevents sperm from getting into vagina and beyond.

Advantages: Easy-to-get form of birth control.

Disadvantages: Can break during sex, so use water-based lubricant, not oil-based. Not only do they weaken condoms, oil-based lubricants can also promote vaginal infections. Must be put on just before intercourse.

Effectiveness: 86 to 97 percent.

Safety issues: Rare, possible allergy to materials or added spermicidal foam.

Diaphragm ($100 to $200 to fit and buy)

What is it? Dome-shaped device that is placed over the cervix. First apply spermicide jelly to outside and inside, then insert through vaginal opening and push into place.

How does it work? Diaphragm holds spermicide against cervix, killing sperm.

Advantages: Only have to use it when you need birth control. Nonhormonal form of birth control.

Disadvantages: Must keep in place for six hours after intercourse. Must use extra contraceptive foam if second intercourse after one to two hours. Can be challenging to learn how to insert. Can dislodge during intercourse. Can be uncomfortable.

Effectiveness: 82 percent.

Safety issues: Minimal. Irritation if sensitive to spermicide.

Cervical Cap ($100 to $200)

What is it? A cap that fits snugly over the cervix. Apply spermicide to inside, then insert.

How does it work? Blocks sperm from entering uterus; spermicide kills any sperm that try.

Advantages: Can be kept in place for up to three days. Only have to use when you need birth control.

Disadvantages: Can be challenging to learn how to insert properly.

Effectiveness: 88 percent.

Safety issues: Minimal. Irritation if sensitive to spermicide.

Sponge: Protectaid-Canada and Today brand-U.S. ($3 each)

What is it? Soft circular foam sponge that is inserted in the vagina so that it covers the cervix.

How does it work? Sponge is saturated with spermicide so it blocks sperm from getting through cervix, kills sperm, and absorbs semen.

Advantages: Can be inserted at an earlier time and left in place. Is effective for up to twelve hours and multiple acts of intercourse.

Disadvantages: Not currently on the market in U.S. Must be left in for six hours after intercourse.

Effectiveness: 90 percent.

Safety issues: Can cause some irritation to cervix if woman is sensitive to spermicide.

Vaginal Contraceptive Film ($0.50 to $3/use)

What is it? Thin film (about the size of a business card) made of spermicide. You use your finger to insert it high in the vagina. Can be inserted from fifteen minutes to one hour prior to intercourse, and cannot be felt by either partner. It dissolves, providing protection.

How does it work? Spermicide kills sperm on contact.

Advantages: Less mess than usual spermicidal foam or jelly.

Disadvantages: Have to insert very close to time of intercourse for it to be effective.

Effectiveness: 96 percent.

Safety issues: Irritation if sensitive to spermicide.

Sterilization: Tubal Ligation (women, $1,000–$2,000), Vasectomy (men, $250–$500)

What is it? Tubal Ligation: Surgical procedure in which the fallopian tubes are both permanently tied off, clipped, or cauterized so that sperm cannot travel inside them and reach the egg. Can be done as outpatient surgery, or after vaginal or cesarean-section delivery. *Vasectomy:* Outpatient surgery (done under local anesthetic) that ties the vasa tubes (that carry the sperm from the testicles to the internal sex organs) so that the sperm can no longer end up in the semen.

How does it work? Permanent blockage of tubes so sperm and egg cannot meet.

Advantages / Disadvantages: This is permanent birth control. Must have surgery. In general, tubal ligation is more complicated and often less effective than vasectomy. There are big differences between a vasectomy and tubal ligation in terms of degree of surgery (vasectomy is a low risk, office-based thirty-minute procedure, while tubal ligation is done in an operating room, usually under general anesthesia, and requires longer recovery time). The cost is also quite different since tubal ligation often costs four times as much as a vasectomy. Tubal ligation has a greater failure rate (especially ten years after) when done in women under the age of thirty, and is possibly less effective if done postpartum immediately after delivery. There is also a small risk of future tubal pregnancies with tubal ligation.

Effectiveness: 99.7 percent. But failure rate for tubal ligation higher than vasectomy.

Safety issues: Risks in any surgery with general anesthesia, risk of bleeding.

Conclusion

Birth control is one of those big issues that nearly every mother has to face until she is postmenopausal. You have many choices of birth control, but the right match depends on your personal needs and medical history as well as your husband's needs and preferences. Consider these factors along with your options as you search for the method best for both of you—so you can freely enjoy your God-given gift of sex!

15

When Getting Pregnant Again Isn't So Easy

"Well, at least you already have a child . . ." If you are one of those mothers struggling to conceive again and have heard this phrase, you can vouch for the fact that this is the *last* thing you want or need to hear. After being so diligent about practicing birth control to avoid getting pregnant at the "wrong time," ironically, many couples face the very frustrating issue of infertility when it is the "right time" to have another child.

> *"What is the best thing I can do to get pregnant? Is there a reason I haven't conceived again?"*

Secondary infertility—the condition of having already had a child and having difficulty getting pregnant after a year of trying—is reportedly more common than being infertile without having had any children. Those of you struggling with secondary infertility probably are having a more difficult time than almost anyone imagines. Many people freely advise that you should just be grateful for the family you already have. That likely leaves you feeling more isolated and downright guilty about your normal, understandable feelings. The desire to have a child, whether it is your first or fifth, is a deep longing that doesn't evaporate easily; rather it spurs a couple on to find solutions. And thankfully, there often *are* solutions.

But first things first. If you aren't having sex often enough during the ripest part of your cycle, then you are less likely to conceive. This is a common factor in secondary infertility since, as we all know, caring for a child or children can sure play havoc with a couple's sex life. Dr. Colleen McNally advises, "If you are trying to get pregnant, we recommend that from the last day of your period to day 20 [of your cycle] that you need to have sex every other day." Others recommend having intercourse every day during the six days before ovulation.[1]

Second, a recent study found that the majority of couples who do not conceive after a year of trying *do* conceive during the second year.[2] So if you increase the frequency of your rendezvous and you are not yet at the end of the second year of trying, the odds are still in your favor.

Miscellaneous Conception Tips

1. Men should wear boxers rather than briefs (heat inside briefs can decrease sperm).
2. Avoid using vaginal lubricants during intercourse (since they may affect sperm).
3. Measure basal body temperature orally (using basal thermometer) every morning and chart results to look for the time of ovulation (temperature drops one to two days before ovulation, then rises for one to two days after ovulation).

Basal Body Temperature: Are You "Hot to Trot"?

Many couples succeed at conceiving because they use the tried-and-true basal body temperature method to help them know when Mom ovulates. This low-cost predictor method requires that you buy a special "basal body thermometer"—which is inexpensive, ultrasensitive, and comes as either a digital or glass type. The thermometer is available at most pharmacies, or online at resources such as ConceptionStore.com. The thermometer comes with the "Basal Body Temperature Chart," and since you need a new chart every month you do this, you can get additional charts either from your ob-gyn or download charts free from many sites (such as BabiesDirect.net at www.kidsdirect.net/BD).

Why is the temperature change important? Because if you will commit to measuring your oral temperature every morning and writing down that temperature each day on the chart, you likely will see right when you ovulate. Typically your basal temperature drops slightly during the day or two days just prior to ovulation, then rises between 0.5 to 1.5 degrees when you ovulate—which means that is when you are likely to be most fertile. So remember, when you're "hot," you're hot-to-trot.

The only catch is, you have to measure your temperature the right way at the right time for it to be an accurate ovulation predictor. It may sound strange, but you need to measure your temperature at the same time each morning, before you get out of bed, or the graph will not be accurate. In fact, it is recommended that before you go to bed at night, shake down the mercury if it is the glass variety and place the thermometer so you can reach it without hardly moving a muscle. Then in the morning, *do not* get out of bed first. Just that little bit of effort of getting out of bed can raise your temperature enough to throw off your graph. Once you have your temperature reading, record it on the chart with the date. The next day, record your temp on the next line over, and so forth. Then watch for the "hot spot."[3]

One other indicator of fertility to watch for is the character of your vaginal discharge. When it is thin, slippery, clear, and the consistency of egg whites, it means ovulation is coming, so you may be more able to conceive. When it is very sticky and thick, the sperm will have a hard time getting through the cervix, and you are not close to ovulation.[4]

Basal Body Temperature (BBT) and Cervical Mucus Chart

Name: Dates: from / / to / /

Cycle Day	1	2	3	4	5	6	7	8	9	10	11	12	13	14	15	16	17	18	19	20	21	22	23	24	25	26	27	28	29	30	31	32	33	34	35	36	37	38	39	40
Weekday																																								
Date/Time																																								
99.1																																								
99.0																																								
98.9																																								
98.8																																								
98.7																																								
98.6																																								
98.5																																								
98.4																																								
98.3																																								
98.2																																								
98.1																																								
98.0																																								
97.9																																								
97.8																																								
97.7																																								
97.6																																								
97.5																																								
97.4																																								
97.3																																								
97.2																																								
97.1																																								
97.0																																								
96.9																																								
Intercourse																																								
Cervical Mucus Type																																								

Cervical Mucus: P= on period, D=dry, M=mucus, E=egg white

Notes: (List any changes to your routine)

Factors in Infertility

Age

The likelihood of getting pregnant is also greatly affected by how old both the woman and man are when trying to conceive. A woman's fertility rate starts to decline when she is 27 years old. The same study that gave us good news about conceiving in the second year of trying also confirmed that fertility decreases as both men and women get older. Only 3 percent of 19- to 26-year-olds, 6 percent of 27- to 34-year-olds, and 9 percent of 35- to 39-year-olds failed to conceive in the second year—provided the male partner was under age 40. The study found that if the woman was 35 to 39, 18 percent of couples did not conceive the first year if the man was younger than 40. That percentage increased to 28 percent not conceiving if the man was over 40. If the woman was 35 to 39 and the man was under 40, only 9 percent did not conceive in the second year. If the man was over 40, 16 percent did not conceive in the second year.[5]

> *"Am I too old to have more children?"*

Dr. McNally confirms that fertility and the risks of pregnancy both change greatly after a woman turns 40: "Fertility dramatically decreases after 40. After 40 the risk of miscarriage is 40 percent, and there is also an increased risk of preterm labor. Plus, the risk of Down's syndrome increases; it is 1 in 190 at age 35 and rises to a risk of 1 in 8 by age 48. But there is [also] a 1 in 200 risk of miscarriage with amniocentesis, so you need to ask yourself what you would do if the results were abnormal—is it worth the risk?"

The Reproductive Medicine Associates of New Jersey studies show that the chance of getting pregnant in any given month declines to approximately 3 percent when women reach the age of 40, and is virtually zero by the time women are 45.[6] According to the Centers for Disease Control, once a woman turns 42, her chances of having a baby using her own eggs is less than 10 percent. By age 42, 90 percent of a woman's eggs are projected to be chromosomally abnormal.[7]

Stress

Stress may be a factor in your fertility, for stress affects the reproductive cycle and can suppress ovulation.[8] The old grandmotherly advice to "just relax and stop trying to get pregnant, and you probably will" has some scientific backing to support it. A study at the Women's Center of the Mind/Body Medical Institute in Boston found that 50 percent of couples (many previously treated extensively for infertility) who took part in a program that combined relaxation-response techniques and stress-management group therapy became pregnant within six months.[9]

"Does stress stop you from conceiving?"

Stress can cause infertility. And if you undergo infertility testing and treatment and find you have infertility issues, it can cause more stress.[10] If you are dealing with infertility now, and especially if you need to proceed with medical testing and intervention, I strongly recommend that you participate in either group counseling, group stress management, and/or personal counseling.

Testing for Fertility

Fertility testing starts with a thorough medical history from both you and your husband. Then several tests are commonly done to help determine if there are any physical reasons that would explain why you and your husband have not been able to conceive. Doctors need to check every aspect of the egg and sperm production process as well as the path they each take to see if there are any roadblocks interfering with the trip of the sperm swimming to the egg. Next they will check to see if the fertilizing of the egg and implanting in the lining of the uterus are happening properly. To accomplish all of this, the testing starts with a pelvic exam for you, measurement of the blood hormone levels in your body, and a check of your basal body temperature when you get up each morning to see if and when you are ovulating. For your spouse, the doctor will order semen specimen analysis to check sperm count and activity of the sperm. To see if a "block" happens when the sperm interacts with your cervical mucus, a postcoital test is usually performed. Your doctor will have you come to the office within twenty-four hours after intercourse so he or she can take a sample of your cervical mucus and then analyze it to see if the sperm can move through it.

Next, to see if the pathway is clear, a hysterosalpingogram X-ray test is done in which a dye is injected through the cervix and watched via X ray to see if there is "smooth sailing" (or should I say, "swimming") up through your uterus to the Fallopian tubes and the egg.

Another test will be done to see if your uterus is cooperating. A small piece of the lining of the uterus is removed for analysis in a test called an endometrial biopsy. This is done to see if the uterine environment is cycling as it should—preparing for implantation, then shedding monthly if you are not pregnant.

Other tests done to check on the reproductive organs in your body may include:

- *Pelvic ultrasound,* a sound-wave test which they also use to see if your ovaries are making eggs normally
- A surgical test called *laparoscopy,* which is done through a small cut in your abdomen; a thin scope with a light is inserted inside your abdomen to look directly at your ovaries and other internal structures to see if cysts, endometriosis, or scar tissue are there and could explain your difficulties with conceiving.[11]

Thanks to these tests and evaluations, causes for infertility can often be found. The most common physical causes of secondary infertility in women include:

- *blocked Fallopian tubes*
- *adhesions* (or bands of scar tissue) *from cesarean section or pelvic infections*—these could be interfering with Fallopian tube function

- *hormonal abnormalities* (such as thyroid or pituitary)
- *problems with ovulation,* which can be from cysts, endometriosis

In men the causes are more commonly lower sperm count, no sperm production, or abnormal functioning of sperm. The age issue, however, is still the most likely cause for infertility in many couples, since it is very common now for couples to start trying for their second baby after Mom has passed age thirty-five.

Got Tests, Need Treatment

How you treat infertility depends on what answers come back with the test results. If you find there is a problem with ovulation, medications can help you produce eggs. If the problem is a blockage in the Fallopian tubes or adhesions, then an option would be to harvest the egg from your ovary, fertilize it outside your womb, then put the embryo into your uterus to implant and grow. What if age is an issue for one or both of you? If you are a woman over forty, it is likely your infertility specialist may recommend using eggs from a donor (who may be someone you know or an anonymous young, healthy woman usually under age thirty). If your husband is older, or found to have a low sperm count or poorly functioning sperm, then sperm from a male donor may be recommended.

Many couples, however, find out that all their tests came out normal—which is good news, yet frustrating since they still have been unable to conceive. Now what? According to Dr. McNally, the best approach is to start with the least invasive treatments and then move toward more invasive treatments if necessary. In other words, start out by helping the natural processes along a little, and see if that bit of help is enough. If not, then consider treatments that get involved with the fertilization and implantation more directly.

A common place to start is with fertility drugs and hormone injections. Clomid and Pergonal are both drugs that cause multiple eggs to "ripen" and release at the same time, while hormone injections such as Gonal-F and Follistim help orchestrate when ovulation occurs. With this treatment alone you increase your chances of at least one egg being fertilized through intercourse in a given cycle. Those sperm must be saying, "So many eggs . . . so little time!" Of course, a side effect of this treatment (as well as others that transfer multiple embryos to the uterus) is that you may get more kids than you bargained for if multiple fertilized eggs implant successfully. Are you prepared for triplets? Or quintuplets?

If either you or your husband is age forty or older, then your infertility doctor may advise skipping some lesser invasive techniques so you can maximize your chances of pregnancy in a shorter amount of time.

Listed below are many of the current approaches to treatment of infertility, in the order that they most likely would be offered. Most couples can be treated successfully with drugs, hormones, surgery, and assisted insemination. Only 5 percent of families currently proceed to in vitro–type options.[12]

Some Current Infertility Treatment Options[13]

Fertility drugs/hormone injections (including Clomid or Pergonal, Gonal-F and Follistim). These are orchestrated together to stimulate the ovaries to produce multiple "ripe" eggs and then control when the eggs are released (ovulation) or harvested.[14]

Intrauterine insemination. This procedure puts a concentrated sample of Dad's washed sperm directly into the uterus to get a higher concentration of sperm into the Fallopian tubes. Often done along with fertility drugs and timed so that the sperm are injected when ovulation is happening so you can increase the chances of fertilization.

Donor semen for intrauterine insemination. This is helpful when there are sperm abnormalities, or if husband previously had a vasectomy.

Selective fertility surgery. When the tests reveal that a mom has abdominal adhesions, a Fallopian tube blockage that can be fixed, or endometriosis, then a specialist may be able to make the problem go away with surgery—and restore fertility.

GIFT: Gamete Intrafallopian Transfer. This procedure helps make the baby by putting the eggs and sperm in the Fallopian tubes at the same time.

Several of Mom-to-be's eggs (or an egg donor's eggs), that were "ripened" using fertility drugs/hormones, are harvested from the ovary (usually using a needle through the wall of the vagina), and then are combined with Dad's sperm sample inside the Fallopian tube. Some have slightly greater success with this method than with in vitro fertilization, possibly because the eggs and sperm are outside the body for a shorter period of time, and because the Fallopian tube is the natural habitat for fertilization to occur.[15]

IVF: in vitro fertilization. This is making babies in a petri dish. Mom-to-be's eggs (harvested from the ovary) are combined with Dad's sperm sample in the petri dish. Then those eggs that are fertilized are allowed to grow into embryos for about three to five days. If there are several embryos produced, then on average two to four are transferred into the uterus. Then it's time to wait. . . . Usually about ten days after the transfer, an in-office pregnancy test is performed. If the test is negative, most couples repeat this procedure. Many infertility centers offer frozen storage of any extra embryos produced in the petri dish, so the mom-to-be doesn't have to go through so much with the next IVF cycle—or in case she wants to get pregnant again in a few years.

Intracytoplasmic sperm injection with in vitro fertilization (ICSI). This is in vitro fertilization with an extra twist (or should I say "shove") because in this technique, the eggs are not left alone with the sperm to do their own thing, but each egg is individually injected with a single sperm. This is especially used when there are very low sperm counts.

Surrogate mother. This is an alternative that some families turn to if Mom cannot physically carry another pregnancy to term; perhaps because of fibroids, a hysterectomy, a cervix that is "incompetent" (cannot hold in the pregnancy), or other medical problems. A surrogate mother carries the fetus in her uterus and may be impregnated through several approaches:

- Surrogate's eggs + intrauterine sperm injection of Dad-to-be's sperm
- In vitro fertilization using either Mom-to-be's eggs, surrogate mother's eggs, or a different donor's eggs + Dad-to-be's sperm or donor sperm

Pick a Winner

Infertility treatment centers are popping up all across the country, so you may have several choices of doctors and centers that are infertility specialists in your area. But check on a few things so you can find the best specialist for your family. Inquire about their success rates and how much experience the doctor(s) have with infertility. Do they offer the range of possible treatments you would personally consider? Are you comfortable there? This is very important since you will have to deal with enough discomfort as it is. Is it close enough to your home? Depending on your treatment, you may have to make trips to the center when the timing is critical, and you don't want to end up stuck in traffic on the highway.

You'll likely want to begin your search by asking your regular ob-gyn physician for a referral to a specialist. But if you need additional help finding a reputable infertility physician in your area, an excellent fertility support organization, RESOLVE, offers reputable referrals to members through their Help Line: 1-888-623-0744, www.resolve.org. One notable reliable network of fertility specialists is Advanced Reproductive Care, Inc. (ARC). This group will advise you of one of their specialists near you if you submit a request on their website: www.arcfertility.com. Many ARC physicians offer a more affordable package deal if you pay up front for fertility treatment.

A Long and Winding Road

The truth behind all this infertility testing and treating is that not only are many of the tests and treatments uncomfortable or physically painful, the whole process can also be psychologically "painful." Since many of the fertility medications and hormone injections can make your emotions fluctuate greatly, it often is an emotionally taxing time. At minimum, the testing and treating is very stressful for both wife and husband. Of course, if the testing reveals a specific reason why you are not yet pregnant, and it is a treatable cause, most parents agree that the tests were worth the discomfort. But you also must be prepared to hear what many couples hear: that "no reason" was found in the testing. Often both husband and wife ride a monthly roller coaster of emotions with new hope at the start of a cycle, then dashed hopes at the end when once again the period comes and pregnancy does not. Many couples become depressed and angry, and some end up separated or divorced after the ordeal of infertility testing and treatment.

Take action to get the personal support and counseling you and your husband need. It is extremely important to take care of your marriage in the midst of this stressful process. When you are in the midst of secondary infertility, you may have to seek professional support and comfort. Since you "already have a child," many friends or family members do not understand how difficult this situation is for you and they may not be very empathetic. The fact that you are newly disappointed each month you do not conceive is one level of sadness and stress, but if you then move on to fertility testing, additional strain and pain are inevitable. If you do not get adequate support from your family or friends, there are excellent support groups (such as RESOLVE) and materials you can turn to.[16]

You need to weather this time together and come to an agreement about how far you will take the testing and fertility treatments. You can never put a price on the value of a child, but infertility testing and especially infertility treatment is very expensive, and usually not covered in full—if at all—by medical insurance. (Currently only twelve states have laws that say insurance must pay for infertility treatments.[17]) You also may be asked to consider fertility treatments that push the boundaries of your personal values and ethics. How far will *you* go? Establish limits that you both mutually agree to before taking any major steps, and agree to reevaluate your limits as time, testing, and treatments go on.

When evaluating why you cannot get pregnant again, the basic thing to keep in mind is that something has changed that is affecting your fertility as a couple, or you were just very blessed to get pregnant so easily the first time. The "something" that has changed may be less frequent intercourse, or more stress in your lives, or an age-related decrease in fertility—especially if you are now over thirty-five. Other things that could have changed are physical ones, such as a decrease in your husband's sperm count or activity, or change in your body since delivery, such as adhesions in your pelvis from surgery, endometriosis scarring, effects from pelvic infection, development of ovarian cysts, or hormonal changes.

The usual approach to treatment is from least invasive to most invasive (unless the mom is over forty), with tough choices and at times rough symptoms along the way. You may feel like you are living under a microscope. In some ways, you are. But the best news is that there are many effective treatments for infertility. Work with your infertility specialist to choose the right ones for you.

My friend, if you are struggling with infertility, I pray you are blessed with morning sickness in the very near future, and with at least one bundle of joy in your arms months later.

16

Those Fluctuating Hormones—From PMS to Perimenopause

Amazingly Feminine

God made each of us who are mothers women first. He gave us amazing hormones and organs that enable life to literally spring from our bodies. But these same hormones are hard to handle when they fluctuate wildly during certain challenging seasons of womanhood—such as puberty, pregnancy, postpartum depression, periods of premenstrual syndrome, and perimenopause. You have likely already been through the first two of these seasons. But now you may be regularly dealing with premenstrual syndrome, and perhaps you'll soon be in perimenopause, that transitional time leading up to menopause.

What are the best ways to cope with these fluctuating hormones? How do we sort out whether what we feel and say is our hormones "talking" or our own true voice?

If you are suffering with premenstrual syndrome (PMS) or the more severe form, premenstrual dysphoric disorder (PMDD), the good news is that the medical profession *knows* it isn't all in your head. Rather we know it's all in your hormones. And we have effective treatment options to offer you. Likewise, if you are enduring the uncomfortable symptoms that can accompany perimenopause, you also have several treatment options available that can help you endure the havoc from these fluctuating hormones.

PMS—"Please Make It Stop!"

I empathize with those of you who suffer with PMS and PMDD. Feeling lousy to downright awful two out of every four weeks is a very difficult way to live. For the two weeks prior to their period, women with PMS can have a combination of physical symptoms such as breast tenderness, headache, lower backache, overall aches and pains, cramping, abdominal bloating, water retention, and weight gain. Plus, these can be accompanied by mental, emotional, and behavioral symptoms such as difficulty thinking or concentrating, depression, anger, irritability, anxiety, crying spells, social withdrawal, and cravings for starchy and salty foods and chocolate. Do these symptoms sound familiar?

> *"PMS is getting worse with age. Is there any relief for me (and my family)?"*

For these symptoms to be "PMS," they must be limited to the two weeks before the period starts and disappear soon after menstruation begins. They must be mild enough so you can still "function," but severe enough to bother you (and possibly those you live with).[1] Many of you live with these symptoms; estimates range from 20 to 50 percent of women. Sometimes it is difficult to sort out what is PMS and what is not, so most doctors recommend you keep a PMS diary and record all the days you feel these symptoms, which symptoms, and when your period occurred and stopped. Then check to see if the symptoms are occurring on days other than the two weeks prior to your period. If so, then it is *not* PMS.

Does PMS get worse as women get older? Dr. Colleen McNally says it does. "It's probably the fluctuation of menstrual hormones that causes it to be worse as women get older." By definition, PMS occurs only when women ovulate. So if you are on birth control pills, you shouldn't have PMS. In fact, that is one of the possible treatments for women who do not respond to other, less drastic treatment measures. But if you find you have these symptoms the first two weeks of each cycle even though you are on the pill, talk with your doctor.

Treatments that help many women include:

- *Change diet*—Decrease or avoid intake of sugars, simple carbohydrates, caffeine, and alcohol during the two weeks prior to your period.
- *Moderate exercise*
- *Stress reduction*
- *Calcium supplement*—"Tums" (1,200 mg per day calcium carbonate) is the only nutritional supplement found to significantly decrease PMS symptoms in a well-controlled clinical study. In this study, 55 percent of women taking calcium had at least a 50 percent improvement in their symptoms, and another 29 percent had at least a 75 percent improvement in their symptoms.[2]
- *Magnesium supplement may be helpful*—Preliminary studies show promising results, but they are not yet conclusive. The supplement may help alleviate mood changes and headache in some women.[3]
- *B-6 supplement may help, but watch the quantity*—Studies are not conclusive that vitamin B-6 helps, even though there has long been the belief that it does. If you wish to use it, do not exceed the upper safety limit of 100 mg per day.[4]
- *No herbals have been shown effective in studies to date*—There were inconsistent results in studies of evening primrose oil.
- *Nonsteroidal anti-inflammatory drugs such as Aleve, naprosyn, ibuprofen*

If your PMS symptoms are still problematic, prescription medications can often help:

- *Zoloft (sertraline)* or *Prozac (fluoxetine)* SSRI antidepressants
- *Diuretics*—to get rid of excess water in body
- *Birth control pills*—to stop ovulation and symptoms
- *Anti-anxiety medications*

If you are one of those who suffer with PMS, I encourage you to keep trying until you find the combination of treatments just right for you.

When Is It PMDD?

Premenstrual Dysphoric Disorder (PMDD) sounds a lot like PMS, but PMS is like a gentle rain shower compared to the hurricane-force symptoms often experienced with PMDD. The mood symptoms must be severe enough to seriously affect your relationships and impair your functioning at work or school for it to be diagnosed as PMDD. The psychiatric criteria for PMDD are as follows (a woman may have PMDD if in the last year she had five or more of the following symptoms during the week before menstruating for most of her menstrual cycles):

- Depression (hopelessness; more than just feeling sad or blue)
- Anxiety (feeling keyed up or on edge)
- Severe mood swings (feeling suddenly sad or extremely sensitive to rejection)
- Anger or irritability
- Decreased interest in usual activities (work, school, friends, hobbies)
- Difficulty concentrating
- Decreased energy
- Appetite changes (overeating or cravings for certain foods)
- Sleep problems (insomnia, early-morning waking, or oversleeping)

- Feeling overwhelmed or out of control
- Physical symptoms, such as bloating, breast tenderness, joint pain, or headaches

The symptoms of PMDD end with menopause, when menstruation stops and the levels of hormones in the body that regulate menstruation no longer rise and fall each month.[5]

Women with PMDD need drug treatment, and the best help seems to come with medications such as Zoloft (sertraline) or Prozac (fluoxetine), both called "selective serotonin reuptake inhibitor antidepressants." The drug named Sarafem is also widely used, but it is actually chemically the same as Prozac. They just gave it another name to earmark it for treatment of PMDD. According to Dr. Colleen McNally, these drugs are given in a different way than is usually prescribed for depression. "These are given at different dosages than the usual for depression. Studies also show they are effective when only given during the two weeks of symptoms." Some women also benefit from the anti-inflammatory drug Ponstel (mefenamic acid) when it is given for the physical symptoms. Women with PMDD also may be helped by making the same lifestyle changes recommended for those with PMS.

There Goes PMS and PMDD, Here Comes Perimenopause

If you currently deal with the uncomfortable symptoms of PMS or PMDD, the good news is that both of these conditions disappear at menopause because they occur only when you are ovulating. The not-so-good news is that as ovulation ceases, there is a five- to ten-year period called *perimenopause* when you may acquire a whole different bunch of temporary, uncomfortable symptoms. Let's look at what these symptoms are and how to relieve them.

Why the Pause for Menopause?

But first, you may be wondering why we are discussing menopause in a book for mothers with young children, especially since many of you will not face this issue for many years. Well, you're right that it will likely be a long time yet, because the average age that perimenopause begins is 47.5, and the average age of menopause is 51.[6] But it turns out, perimenopause can start in women during their late 30s (it is a 10-year range), and since many moms are having their first children after the age of 30, quite a few of you *will* face this issue soon. Plus, in the MOPS survey many asked for the scoop on menopause and especially wanted the latest info on hormone replacement therapy. So here it is.

You have arrived at menopause after you have gone one year without having a menstrual period. But there is quite a hormone ride on the journey between the start of perimenopause and the menopause finish line. In perimenopause, many hormones are fluctuating, but the most significant hormone fluctuation is a major drop in estrogen levels. It is no wonder perimenopause sometimes feels like you've just crested a hill on a roller coaster and now are zooming straight down. In a sense, that is what your hormones are doing. And the symptoms of perimenopause can be very hard to cope with.

Between 70 and 85 percent of perimenopausal women experience uncomfortable symptoms including hot flashes, night sweats, sleep problems, mood swings, memory impairment, trouble thinking, vaginal dryness, increased urinary tract symptoms, and irregular periods leading up to their final menstrual period.[7]

The good news is that these symptoms do go away and usually are mild when they start. But they intensify until you reach the midpoint (which usually is when you have your last menstrual period). Then the symptoms decrease gradually until the "change" is finished. Most of these uncomfortable symptoms are directly related to the decrease in estrogen levels and the change in other hormone levels. Menopause also marks the point in time when a woman becomes more at risk for serious health conditions such as osteoporosis, high cholesterol, and coronary heart disease, again because her body's estrogen levels have greatly declined.

So it makes sense that if you put back the estrogen, then the symptoms and bad effects of menopause will decrease, right? And that is exactly why countless numbers of women have taken replacement estrogen. To decrease the risk of uterine cancer from the replacement of estrogen, women have been put on a combination of two hormones, estrogen and progesterone, rather than estrogen alone. The usual term for this dynamic duo is hormone replacement therapy (or HRT). It is estimated that between 8 million and 16 million women over fifty are currently on HRT.[8]

To Take Hormones or Not to Take Hormones? The New Question

Recently a major change occurred in the recommendation of hormone replacement therapy. It is no longer a question of *when* you should start hormone replacement therapy (HRT), but *if* you should take it. New research findings have unearthed some risks with HRT. Until July 2002, medical research seemed to support the theory that taking HRT as a long-term treatment was not only pretty safe but actually might decrease the rate of heart attacks and decrease osteoporosis. The previous research showed that women on long-term hormone therapy had a slightly higher risk of getting breast cancer, but it was believed that the reduction in heart attacks far outweighed the risk of getting breast cancer.

> *"At what age should I start thinking about taking replacement hormones?"*

But in July 2002, worrisome five-year study results were released from a huge women's health study done through the National Institutes of Health, called the WHI study (Women's Health Initiative). The results showed that there was an increased risk of heart attacks, blood clots, and strokes in those women on HRT, in addition to the already suspected increase in the risk of breast cancer. What kind of increase are we talking about? The WHI study found that in a usual year, heart attacks hit 37 of every 10,000 Prempro users in the study, versus 30 out of 10,000 placebo users. The annual stroke rate rose from 21 to 29 per 10,000, and the breast-cancer rate increased from 30 to 38 per 10,000.

Why are these study results so different from results of previous studies? The previous studies did show that women who were on hormones were less likely to have heart disease, but the way these previous studies were designed, they did not account for the fact that the women who decided to take hormones were already healthier than the general population of women. It only looked like the hormones deserved the credit. This most recent study solved that issue by putting all sorts of women on the hormones and watching their health over five years. One of the criticisms of these new study findings is that it included women up to the age of seventy-nine, which in itself may increase the risk of heart attacks.

Where does that leave the thousands of women who suffer with perimenopause symptoms? Hormonal therapy still is the most effective way to quiet the symptoms of menopause. Does this mean all women should avoid HRT? Our expert, Dr. Colleen McNally, offers this advice: "In review of the Women's Health Initiative study results, I feel that there are several important issues to consider. To date, there does not appear to be increased risks in heart attacks and breast cancer in patients who are taking estrogen only. Therefore, it is possible that the effects we are seeing are due solely to the Provera (progesterone) component of the hormone replacement therapy.

"There does appear to be a small increased risk of breast cancer in women who are taking Prempro as compared to those women who are not . . . and we know that in some women there is an increased risk of stroke and thromboembolic events with hormone replacement therapy. The unanswered question was whether or not there is an increased incidence of heart attacks. [But] the study did show decreased risks of hip fractures and colorectal cancer in the women taking Prempro.

"The question is where do we go from here? I still believe that a woman's decision whether or not to take hormone replacement therapy is a very personal decision and needs to be individualized to each patient. It truly depends on the menopausal symptoms that you are experiencing and the severity of those symptoms. It also depends on your personal assessment of your future risks for osteoporosis, colorectal cancer, cardiovascular disease, and breast cancer."[9]

Menopause Treatment Alternatives

There are a few choices to consider that may be lower in risk.

Short-Term HRT. One issue seems to be how long a woman takes HRT. Although it may seem like contradictory advice, the WHI study did not show the same kinds of risks for women when HRT was used for less than five years. If a woman has debilitating symptoms of menopause, such as hot flashes, night sweats, insomnia, mood swings, and memory loss, many experts agree now that less than five years is the magic time frame. The sooner women can stop the treatment, the better.

Lower Dose Estradiol with Prometrium. Another option is to take lower doses of these two hormones, and in forms that more closely resemble our natural hormones. The usual HRT treatment called Prempro is a combination of a fairly high dose (0.625 mg) Premarin estrogen (obtained from the urine of pregnant horses) and synthetic progesterone. An alternative would be a lower dose of estradiol and the progesterone Prometrium or micronized progesterone.[10] But Dr. McNally points out that "it would be premature to say that other forms of progestins such as norethindrone or micronized progesterone are better than Provera, as those have yet to be studied with such a large number of patients."

Other Medications. Depending on your menopausal symptoms, there are a number of other medications that may take care of your specific need without HRT. Dr. McNally says, "Hot flashes can be difficult to manage. However, we have had some success with medications used to treat depression and hypertension. The treatment of vaginal dryness can be helped with locally applied estrogen that is not systemically absorbed. Nonhormonal medications can be used to combat osteoporosis. Cholesterol-lowering drugs appear to be very effective in decreasing one's risk for a heart attack."

Nutritional and Herbal Supplements. The common thread among many of the dietary supplements is that many contain estrogen-like compounds called "phytoestrogens" or "isoflavones." These compounds are not estrogen, but they appear to balance out the hormones when they are out of whack through the time known as perimenopause.

Soy Food Products. These are a good choice. Asian women report far fewer hot flashes and other symptoms in menopause. Many researchers have suspected that it is related to all the soy food in their daily diet, which can be as high as six servings a day. Isoflavones are known to be present in high amounts in soy foods,[11] and countless numbers of women say they find relief from hot flashes if they eat large amounts of soy foods.[12] Edamame boiled soybeans (1 cup per day) are a great way to bring soy into your daily diet. Another excellent source of soy is the tasty Revival brand soy foods.[13] One serving of Revival gives you 17 grams (bars) or 20 grams (drink) of nongenetically modified, nonchemically processed soy protein and 160 mg of natural isoflavones, which is the same amount that would be in six usual servings of soy (available at www.revivalsoy.com or 1-800-500-2055).

Soy Supplements of Isoflavones. These are not recommended. Studies show that isoflavone supplements taken without soy protein can be harmful to your health. Specifically, they may promote the growth of tumors.

Black Cohosh (Remifemin and Cimicifuga racemosa). This may be effective. It is the most studied herbal choice. The well-tested and standardized brand is Remifemin. A recent review of eight German studies that used Remifemin on menopausal women found that the extract is both safe and effective in reducing the symptoms of menopause, with 80 percent of patients noting a significant reduction in their symptoms within four weeks. Some had a complete disappearance of symptoms after six to eight weeks.[14] The downside is there still are no good studies on long-term safety, and since it may contain plant estrogens, there is concern about its effect on uterus and breast cancer risks. Experts currently suggest not taking it for more than six months.[15] The recommended dose is 40 mg per day.

Red Clover (Promensil). This is not shown to be effective. Even though red clover contains isoflavones, a recent review of the medical literature showed no evidence that red clover decreased hot flashes or other symptoms.[16]

Dong Quai. Findings are not conclusive. University of California San Francisco has done randomized studies on dong quai and found that when used alone, dong quai does not produce estrogen-like responses. It was no more helpful than a placebo in relieving menopausal symptoms.[17] Other studies have suggested that when dong quai is combined with other herbs there may be some relief of menopausal symptoms.

Wild Yam. This is not recommended. Health-food stores carry creams with wild yam in them. Such products say they will deliver natural progesterone hormone through the skin when you rub them on. But the body cannot convert this to human progesterone, and we cannot be certain what is really in these creams.[18]

Hormonal Roller-Coaster Rides

PMS, PMDD, and perimenopause are unpleasant hormonal roller-coaster rides for many women, but there are many treatment options that can help smooth out the wild dips and curves.

More than a few women taking these unpleasant rides have wondered, *Why did God do this to us?* I do not know the answer to that one, but I do know that if I had to choose between the chance to grow and bear a child or the chance to be free from these times of hormone fluctuations, I would still choose the deal I have. How about you?

Another result of hormonal fluctuations is postpartum depression and "baby blues." Let's look at these common mommy mental health issues in the next chapter.

17

Mom's Mental Health—Feeling Blue Rather Than Tickled Pink

"Why are you so sad? You have so much to be thankful for!" "Cheer up! Life's not that bad!" These are well-meaning comments, but when you are fighting depression, life really *is* "that bad." You cannot cheer up or think positively or "pull yourself up by the bootstraps" and make the sadness go away. With depression it often feels like a visitor has moved in permanently, one who torments you day after day. And night after night you may be forced to face these torments while others in your house sleep—yet you cannot.

> *My soul is in anguish. How long, O Lord, how long?—Psalm 6:3*

Living with depression is like trying to do all your usual duties in the dark. Everything takes more effort. And even with your best effort, many things cannot be done the way you could do them if you had some light to work by. There is nothing "light" about depression. It is as if a boulder has suddenly appeared inside the core of your body and is weighing you down with every step and thought you try to put forth. Humor rarely penetrates the fortress that depression builds. People around you can't understand why you just don't find things funny anymore.

Depression is real, painful, and, at times, so horrible to live with that some people are willing to die to make it go away. This choice to die is not that surprising to those who have ever been terribly depressed, because they know this is no way to live. Every day a multitude of moms continue to live with depression while trying to be the very best moms they can be, and depression makes that job many times more difficult. Depression makes it hard to believe you are doing the right things for your child because you know deep down that if you weren't depressed you could be a better mother. Then the guilt really sets in, with feelings such as "my child deserves so much more than I can give," and "I am probably harming my child emotionally because I'm so depressed." These common thoughts just make matters worse.

How Common Is Depression?

According to the National Institute of Mental Health, 12.4 million women in the U.S. are affected by a depressive disorder every year, which translates to 12 percent of all women. Half of those women suffer with a major depressive disorder each year, which means the depression is serious enough to require medication to resolve or relieve it.[1]

What Are the Signs of Depression?

Most people who are depressed have at least several of the following symptoms:

- Sadness, unhappiness, tearfulness
- Sleeping excessively or being unable to sleep (even though you are not being awakened by someone or something else)
- Loss of energy
- Loss of interest in things you previously enjoyed
- Irritability

- Difficulty thinking or concentrating
- Sudden change in appetite
- Physical discomfort
- Feelings of worthlessness
- Thoughts of suicide or death

With major depression, the sufferer would likely have at least five of these symptoms present most of the day, nearly every day, for two weeks or more.[2]

You Feel This Way for a Reason

Although I'm sure poet Elizabeth Barrett Browning never wrote, "How did I get depressed—let me count the ways . . . ," there are unfortunately scores of moms who know this sonnet by heart. When you feel depressed there is a good reason for it. It is a "red flag" signaling that something is not right in your world, and you need to pay attention to the signal. But the "something not right" varies widely from situational reasons to biochemical causes. Some of the common reasons include:

- *Hormone shifts.* This occurs right after childbirth, with PMS, PMDD, and perimenopause.
- *Biochemical imbalance.* Depletion of brain chemicals frequently causes depression.
- *Prone to winter depression (known as S.A.D.: Seasonal Affective Disorder).* When sunlight levels drop, these women become depressed unless treated with light therapy.
- *Sheer exhaustion.* The job of parenting is hard and constant and exhausting, which can make anyone depressed at times.
- *Unresolved anger turned inward.* If you are not dealing with situations that make you angry, and the anger that results, there is a danger of depression.
- *Your needs are not being met.* From sleep deprivation and other physical needs to emotional, mental, and spiritual needs, you are at risk for depression when these aren't met.

- *Issues from your own childhood emerge when you become a parent.*
- *Your situation is not matching your expectations.*

Mild depression that is situational is very often an indicator that you need to work through a conflict and either accept the changes in your situation that are making you angry or depressed, or find a way to change the situation. Once you take either of these actions, the mild depression often lifts. This may be accomplished by talking with your husband, friends, or family. Often we can find hope, practical solutions, and a better ability to cope through their care and counsel. Or you may benefit most from seeing a Christian counselor who understands the pressures and changes you are experiencing; such a person can help you sort through what you can and cannot change.

A Biochemical Imbalance Is Not Your Fault

There still circulates a faulty notion that a woman who is depressed has sinned, or is too emotionally weak, or her faith is too weak so she has brought depression on herself. Or, in other words, if you have depression, it is your own fault. This is not true. Of course, if you willfully disobey God's laws, depression can be a natural consequence to your deliberate sin. But moderate to severe depression—known as major depression—usually results from a biochemical imbalance in the brain that is not related to lack of faith, sin, or emotional weakness. This biochemical imbalance, which is a deficiency of the brain chemical serotonin, needs correction so that a woman can feel and act like herself again. This is exactly what antidepressant medications do; they increase the amount of serotonin the brain cells are exposed to.

Roadblocks to Treatment

Depression is a common problem for moms, yet many do not seek treatment or are inadequately treated. In part this is because it can be hard for a mom to recognize how depressed she is. Many moms also feel ashamed that they feel depressed—they think others might think less of them if they knew about the depression. So the moms hide it. These moms are afraid to ask for help and often they try to "tough it out," which at minimum causes them to suffer more or may even make the depression much worse and harder to treat. Particularly in the church, we need to be clear with one another that depression is very common and happens for very real reasons, and it needs to be treated. Let's each do our part to erase the shame from the diagnosis of depression.

When you have a mental health problem that needs treatment with medication, it is not a sign of failure. Sometimes well-meaning Christians push others to not take medication for mental health issues. But I join many Christian mental health experts, such as Dr. Paul Meier of the Christian Minirth-Meier New Life Mental Health Clinics, in saying that we believe in medication as a help from God for those with depression and anxiety conditions.[3]

The book *Mood Swings* by noted Christian counselors and doctors Paul Meier, Stephen Arterburn, and Frank Minirth is an excellent resource for understanding how brain chemistry influences our moods and emotions, as well as how to find better emotional balance.[4] These mental health experts are the founders of the highly helpful Minirth-Meier New Life Clinics, a group of Christian mental health clinics located throughout the nation. These are places where Christians can go for caring day treatment and inpatient mental health care. For information, call 1-800-NEW-LIFE (1-800-639-5433), or visit their website at www.newlife.com.[5]

Postpartum Depression

One of the most common types of major depression in women is postpartum depression, occurring after delivery in up to 13 percent of women, which translates to a half-million women in the U.S. every year. Postpartum depression is different from "baby blues," which nearly all moms get during the ten days after delivery. According to Dr. Colleen McNally, "Baby blues happens to about 80 percent of moms, and is a few days of tearfulness, feeling overwhelmed, and the feeling of, 'Why am I crying when I'm so happy?' Postpartum depression is when these symptoms last much longer, or are more severe." Dr. McNally says that often the mom is the last to realize she has postpartum depression. According to Dr. McNally, new fathers need to be alert for the symptoms of postpartum depression. In addition to the usual symptoms of depression (as listed above), specific symptoms seen with postpartum depression usually appear in the first four to twelve weeks after delivery and last more than two to three weeks, often over six months.

Why Does Postpartum Depression Happen?

It is believed that the sudden drop in reproductive hormone levels right after delivery is what prompts these mood problems to appear in susceptible women.[6] "Susceptible" women appear to be affected by this decrease in hormones differently than other women. Studies show that one factor that may predict susceptibility is if women have a previous history of depression or a family history of mood disorders.[7] Studies also show that the likelihood of postpartum depression does *not* appear to be related to a woman's educational level, whether her infant is male or female, whether or not she breastfeeds, the type of delivery, or whether or not the pregnancy was planned.[8]

Treating Postpartum Depression

Once a woman is diagnosed with postpartum depression, treatment must begin as soon as possible. The most often prescribed medications in this type of depression are the serotonin reuptake-inhibitor antidepressants Zoloft (sertraline) and Prozac (fluoxetine). Good results are seen in most cases with either drug. Moms must not stop either medication abruptly, but must continue taking it as the doctor recommends or until he or she tells you to taper off the dose. The medication needs to be continued for a minimum of six months beyond the point when the symptoms have gone away.

One major issue for moms with postpartum depression is the fact that if a mom needs to begin antidepressant medication immediately, her doctor may recommend that breastfeeding cease. Because they want to continue breastfeeding, this prompts a lot of moms to try to "tough it out" without starting medication.

In most cases, this is a bad idea. I speak from experience, moms. You may be tough, but it usually isn't worth the sacrifice of not becoming mentally healthier for the hope that your child will be physically healthier from breastfeeding. When I developed postpartum depression after my son was born, I tried to tough it out and refused to start medication so I could breastfeed. Another reason I refused was, in part, because I didn't want to *need* medication. Many months later, when I was mentally and emotionally depleted, I finally agreed to start medication. Because I had waited so long, it took a lot longer to get the depression under control. But once I no longer looked at everything through the dark cloud of depression, life was amazingly different. I now see that it would have been better if I had given up breastfeeding earlier so I could have given my son, my husband, and myself a wife and mother who was more intact.

If you do stop breastfeeding to go on medication for your depression, honor your need to grieve the loss of breastfeeding. It may seem you are compounding your depression with more sadness and depression, but if you let yourself feel the understandable feelings of sadness and loss, you likely will find that they decrease fairly soon. If you try to stuff down these feelings and pretend they don't exist, in the long run you will likely suffer more.

Postpartum Psychosis—An Emergency!

It is nearly impossible to imagine how a mother could believe that killing her two-week-old baby was the right thing to do, yet the small proportion of women who develop postpartum psychosis truly suffer such delusions. Usually this develops within the first two weeks after delivery, and moms who have this may have extreme disorganization of thought, bizarre beliefs and behavior, delusions, and hallucinations.[9] The incidence of suicide and infanticide is extremely high for mothers with postpartum psychosis.

THIS IS A PSYCHIATRIC EMERGENCY. If you know a mom who has recently delivered who is exhibiting any bizarre behavior, please do not wait to get help. This mom and baby may both be in great danger. If you want more information about postpartum depressive disorders, contact Postpartum Support at www.postpartum.net or call 1-805-967-7636.

Common Crunch Times for Depression

There are certain times when moms commonly experience mild to moderate depression. Such times may be completely situation related, or situation as well as biochemically caused. Let's highlight some of these crunch times so you can be on special lookout for your mental and physical health during these times:

- *Postpartum.* After having a baby, every mom needs time to rejuvenate and recover, and all need help at home. Don't turn down the offers of meals. Ask for help and then accept it.
- *Around the holidays.* Though certainly it is a time we all look forward to, the holiday equation is high expectations + excited children + stress factors = *major* energy drain. Try to adjust your expectations and help others know what your limits are during this time.
- *Job change or job loss.* This can be a very stressful time, so take good care of yourself.

Other Helpful "Antidepressants"

To help yourself weather a time of depression, here are some things you can do:

Get counseling. Some women only need to talk with friends and family members to resolve their mild depression, but for moderate to severe depression, I strongly recommend counseling by a qualified Christian counselor, therapist, or psychiatrist. Even when medication is required, counseling still plays a very important role in healing.

Do some aerobic exercise. Studies show that regular aerobic exercise (such as walking on a treadmill for thirty minutes) can improve even cases of moderate to severe depression that have not been helped by medication.[10]

Exercise your faith. A wealth of studies have been done in the last ten years that look at the effects of practicing your faith. Scientists confirm how important exercising your faith is to your mental and physical health: "A recent systematic review of research on religion and health has found a consistent relationship between religion and better mental health. There also appears to be a relationship between religious involvement and better physical health, although the mechanism for this effect is poorly understood."[11] Brain scans with MRI done during meditation and prayer show changes in the brain consistent with relaxation and a better emotional state. It is proposed that we are "hardwired" to communicate with God.[12]

When you feel depressed and overwhelmed, cling to God. Remember that you are not alone, for "The Lord himself goes before you and will be with you; he will never leave you nor forsake you. Do not be afraid; do not be discouraged" (Deuteronomy 31:8). Pray in the midst of it all. Tell God exactly how you feel; he can take it. Read your Bible daily and attend church and Bible study meetings as often as possible. And ask others to pray for you and with you. God offers real hope in seemingly hopeless times. You can lean on that assurance.

Eat and sleep to be merry. You need to care for your physical needs to prevent and treat depression. That includes eating a healthy diet and getting the sleep you need. Moms who are sleep deprived often are also depressed. In fact, a recent study found that 25 percent of new moms who were very sleep deprived also scored high on depression tests. But moms in this study who took naps when baby slept or had partners who took some of the night feedings were less sleep deprived and less likely to be depressed.[13] When you are sleep deprived, sleep is what you need. Take naps. Ask for help so you can get the sleep you are lacking—for everyone's sake.

Do whatever makes you laugh. Laughter truly is one of the best medicines.

Practice gratitude. How we think does affect how we feel (although in cases of moderate to severe depression, "happy thoughts" usually cannot correct the biochemical imbalance). But with mild depression, you can improve your coping by actively choosing to find what you can be grateful for right at that moment. You need not be a Pollyanna and pretend everything is sweetness and light, but truthful searching and honestly saying what you are grateful for can help immensely.

Natural Remedies for Depression

The overall consensus about most natural supplements taken for depression and anxiety is that research studies do not find them reliably helpful, and often they can be hazardous to your health.

Saint John's wort (hypericum). Saint John's wort is clearly the best of the bunch of natural remedies, but studies have not found it to be reliably helpful when one is suffering from moderate to severe depression. A recent randomized clinical trial found that the herb was not any more effective than a sugar pill when given for major depression.[14] Studies of folks with mild depression have suggested it may help. Be careful about self-treating your depression with this herb, for you may be under treated. The most crucial thing to know about Saint John's Wort is that it has dangerous interactions with other medications, such as birth control pills, the blood thinner Coumadin, the transplant drug Cyclosporin, and other antidepressant medications (particularly SSRI-type drugs such as Prozac).

Kava-kava: DANGER. May cause liver disease in users! This herb has become popular because of its calming effect, but recently, at least thirty cases of severe liver damage were connected to kava in Germany, so several European countries have banned the herb.[15] The FDA has also received reports of serious reactions.

Take Care, My Friend

Depression is serious and very painful to endure. Since it is common among women for so many different reasons, it is likely you have or will endure episodes in your adult life. Please take extra good care of yourself, especially in this season of your life as a mom, and remember, there is no shame in being depressed. It is only a "shame" if you do not get the help you need.

Conclusion: Begin Today

How can I be whole—physically, mentally, and spiritually? This one question sums it all up, doesn't it? We want to be whole. Deep down, that is what we all want and seek. But how can we be whole when we are pulled in so many directions? My friend, I'm with you down in the trenches of motherhood. I will be the first to agree with you that motherhood is not easy. You want to do your best—be your best—for your family and your Lord.

Thankfully none of us is called to the job of motherhood and expected to do it alone. God is right with you all the time. And since he is there with you, he knows all the details of your life and your personal struggles. He wants you to talk freely with him about all of it, the good and the bad. You probably don't have the luxury of long stretches of unscheduled time to spend solely in fellowship with God, but you do have free access to God any and every moment of the day or night. Remember this especially in those times when you are trying to get dinner ready and the children are squabbling and then the phone rings and you just want to scream.

> *"How can I be whole—physically, mentally, and spiritually?"*

Remember that God is there for you. He can handle your telling him exactly how you feel, even those times when you just want to scream. He is happy to hear even the briefest prayers, when all you can muster is *"Help."* But he is best able to help us be the women, the mothers, the *everything,* that we are and want to be when we decide to invite him into every aspect of our lives. We must focus on God in the good times as well as the overwhelming times of life. We must admit to ourselves and to God that we cannot do this without him. These are the first real steps to truly taking care of yourself—your *whole* self—and your family the way God intended.

The greatest commandments, according to Jesus Christ, are, "'Love the Lord your God with all your heart and with all your soul and with all your mind.' This is the first and the greatest commandment. And the second is like it: 'Love your neighbor as yourself'" (Matthew 22:37–39). But if you are to care for "others as yourself," how good is that care if you aren't giving yourself good care? In other words, we are called to love and care for ourselves—and care for others—with the same intensity.

It is difficult sometimes to find the right balance, isn't it? That is why I challenge you to take the first step toward caring for yourself today. Be sure you have invited God along with you for every phase of this journey. If you have never done this before, it is very simple to do. Take a moment and pray—which just means that you talk to God—saying, "Lord Jesus, I need you. I cannot do this alone and I know I fall short of what you want me to do and be. Please forgive me and come into my heart. Thank you that you will stay and help me every day. Amen."

If you have prayed this prayer for the first time, you need to tell someone about it. Please contact your pastor at your local church, or your local MOPS leader. They can help you get started with Bible study and fellowship that will help you grow both as a new Christian and as a mother. For other resources to help you in mothering or to find a MOPS group near you, contact the MOPS International office at 1-303-733-5353, email at info@mops.org, or online at www.mops.org.

As we have learned, energy is the commodity that every mother needs, and most moms find they need more energy than they have. In part, this is because stress, particularly emotional stress, is nearly unavoidable for mothers. We care, then "life" happens, so we stress, then we feel exhausted.

That's the cycle. Fortunately, though stress may be unavoidable, it *is* manageable. I challenge you to begin implementing the solutions to stress that we looked at in this book. You can also find good advice in the other books I recommend. Or find a stress management group or seminar in the town where you live.

Exercise is perhaps the most effective stress management tool we have. It directly energizes us. Exercise makes us burn more calories, which helps us manage our weight, build muscle, and improve the fitness of our heart and body physiology. So if you are not already exercising regularly, accept my challenge and begin today.

There is so much you can do to chart a healthy course for your life. Wise eating choices, wise weight-loss approaches, wise lifestyle choices, and proper precautions against the sun and common parental injuries will take you a long way on that course. Another key to protecting your health is making sure you have regular dental and medical checkups including screening for medical conditions that are all too common in women. It is not selfish to take care of yourself, for in taking care of your health *you are* caring for your family. *Your health matters!*

God made you a woman, and with that gift of female chemistry come some interesting challenges, such as PMS, a fluctuating libido, and perimenopause. It is your privilege to carry and give birth to babies, but along with that privilege may come the pain of postpartum depression or the heartbreak and stress when the pregnancy you want is just not happening. I empathize with each of you who are dealing with these challenges.

Dear mom, it is time to start taking better care of yourself. You will have more energy, a better outlook, and be a better mom. And most importantly, you will be more able to serve God in the unique ways he wants for you. I wish you a joyful journey!

> Now to him who is able to do immeasurably more than all we ask or imagine, according to his power that is at work within us, to him be glory in the church and in Christ Jesus throughout all generations, for ever and ever!
>
> Ephesians 3:20–21

CMDA Statement on Hormonal Contraception and Abortion

The Christian Medical & Dental Associations (CMDA) holds firmly that God is the Creator of life, that life begins at conception, and that all human life is of infinite value. We support measures to protect life from its earliest beginnings.

CMDA recognizes that there are differing viewpoints among Christians regarding the broad issue of birth control and the use of contraceptives. The issue at hand, however, is whether or not hormonal birth control methods have post-conceptional effects (i.e., cause abortion). CMDA has consulted many experts in the field of reproduction who have reviewed the scientific literature. While there are data that cause concern, our current scientific knowledge does not establish a definitive causal link between the routine use of hormonal birth control and abortion. However, neither are there data to deny a post-conceptional effect.

Because this issue cannot be resolved with our current understanding, CMDA calls upon researchers to further investigate the mechanisms of action of hormonal birth control. Additionally, because the possibility of abortive effects cannot be ruled out, prescribers of hormonal birth control should consider informing patients of this potential factor.

We recognize the difficulties of providing informed consent while handicapped by lack of definitive information. However, counseling of patients may simply involve asking if they have concerns about potential post-conceptional effects of these methods of birth control. In cases where concern exists, an explanation may follow that includes the known mechanisms of action (e.g., inhibition of ovulation and decreased sperm penetration), as well as the concern about the unanswered question of whether hormones negatively affect the very early stages of life.

CMDA respects and defends the right of our colleagues to refuse to prescribe hormonal birth control when they do so with the concern of a post-conceptional effect.

We recognize that scientific reasoning is not the only factor that influences opinions about the use of hormonal birth control. But, while additional investigation is needed, current knowledge does not confirm or refute conclusions that routine use of hormonal birth control causes abortion. CMDA will continue to monitor new developments.

November 2000

Notes

Yes! Mom's Health Matters!

1. Lisa Delaney, "Women in Motion: What got you moving in the right direction, healthwise?" *Health,* July–August 2001, 94–106.
2. Ibid., excerpt from Sandi Salera Lloyd, 103.

Chapter 1. Your Personal Energy Crisis

1. Bryant and Zick, *Child Rearing Time by Parents: A Report of Research in Progress,* part of Consumer Close-Up series by Cornell's College of Human Ecology; includes data from the 1975–81 "Time Use Longitudinal Panel Study," the 1977–78 "Eleven State Time Use Survey," and the 1985 "Americans Use of Time Data," available online at www.news.cornell.edu.
2. Jean Fleming, *A Mother's Heart* (Colorado Springs: Navpress, 1996), 26.
3. Ibid., 27.
4. *Where's the Sleep? The 1999 Survey of Ohio's Working Families,* University of Cincinnati E-briefs, available online at www.uc.edu/news/ebriefs/momeb .htm, accessed 14 April 2000.

Chapter 2. Stress and Anxiety Reduction for Moms on the Run

1. Elisa Morgan and Carol Kuykendall, *Real Moms: Exploding the Myths of Motherhood* (Grand Rapids: Zondervan, 2002), 15. Reprinted by permission from Zondervan.
2. Ibid., taken from the back cover.
3. Ibid., 18.
4. Ibid., 17–18.
5. Florence Littauer and Marita Littauer, *Getting Along with Almost Anybody* (Old Tappan, N.J.: Revell, 1998). Information used by permission of Florence Littauer, Marita Littauer, and Fleming H. Revell Company.
6. Personal interview with Marita Littauer, President of CLASServices, Inc., 21 November, 2001.

7. Tiffany Field et al., "Stress Is a Noun! No, a Verb! No, an Adjective!" in *Stress and Coping* (Mahwah, N.J.: Lawrence Erlbaum, 1985), 17.
8. E. S. Epel et al., "Stress and body shape: Stress-induced cortisol secretion is consistently greater among women with central fat," *Psychosomatic Medicine* 62, no. 5 (September–October 2000): 623–32.
9. P. M. Peeke and G. P. Chrousos, "Hypercortisolism and obesity," *Annals of the New York Academy of Sciences* 771 (29 December 1995): 665–76.
10. Adapted from Bernd Harmsen's "Progressive Muscle Relaxation," (Stuttgart, Germany), available online at ourworld.compuserve.com/homepages/har/relax.htm, accessed 21 March 2003.
11. Field et al., *Stress and Coping,* 17–18.
12. *Mom's Devotional Bible: NIV* (Grand Rapids: Zondervan, 1996).
13. Elisa Morgan, *Meditations for Mothers: Moments with God Amidst a Busy Nest* (Grand Rapids: Zondervan, 1999).
14. The booklets are $1 each, available from Peale Center for Christian Living, Dept. 5312, 39 Seminary Hill Road, Carmel, NY 10512-1999.
15. Julie Morgenstern, *Organizing from the Inside Out* (New York: Henry Holt, 1998).
16. S. E. Taylor et al., "Biobehavioral responses to stress in females: Tend and befriend, not fight-or-flight," *Psychological Review* 107, no. 3 (July 2000): 411–29.
17. L. S. Berk et al., "Neuroendocrine and stress hormone changes during mirthful laughter," *American Journal of the Medical Sciences* 298, no. 6 (December 1989): 390–96.
18. Excerpt from *MOMSense,* 8 August 2002 episode "Writer at Work," broadcast by Elisa Morgan of MOPS International, available online at www.mops.org. Printed by permission from author Lori Walker.
19. Julia Cameron, "The Basic Tools," in *The Artist's Way: A Spiritual Path to Higher Creativity* (New York: Jeremy P. Tarcher/Putnum, member of Penguin Putnam, 1992), 9–18.

Chapter 3. Healthy Diet—Fueling Your Daily Mom-a-Thon

1. Adelle Davis (1904–74), Food Reference, available online at www.foodreference.com, accessed 24 March 2003.
2. Silva I. Dos Santos et al., "Lifelong vegetarianism and risk of breast cancer: A population-based case-control study among South Asian migrant women living in England," *International Journal of Cancer* 99, no. 2 (10 May 2002): 238–44.

3. C. S. Johnston and D. L. Bowling, "Stability of ascorbic acid in commercially available orange juices," *Journal of the American Dietetic Association* 102, no. 4 (April 2002): 525–29.
4. A. M. Strack et al., "A hypercaloric load induces thermogenesis but inhibits stress responses in the SNS and HPA system," *American Journal of Physiology* 272, no. 3, pt. 2 (March 1997): R840–48; Dorothy Foltz-Gray, "The Relaxing Way to Lose Weight," *Health,* May 2001, 93.
5. "Keen on Beans: A New Soy Label," *UC Berkeley Wellness Letter,* February 2000, 2.
6. Soy milk beverages rated for taste by Consumer Reports in *Consumer Reports Magazine,* February 2002, 8.
7. Deborah Madison, *This Can't Be Tofu!* (New York: Broadway Books, Random House, 2000).
8. S. L. Connor and W. E. Connor, "Are fish oils beneficial in the prevention and treatment of coronary artery disease?" *American Journal of Clinical Nutrition* 66, no. 4 supplement (October 1997): 1020S–31S; I. Bairati et al., "Effects of fish oil supplement on blood pressure and serum lipids in patients treated for coronary artery disease," *Canadian Journal of Cardiology* 8, no. 1 (January–February 1992): 41–46.
9. Penny Kris-Etherton et al., "High-monounsaturated fatty acid diets lower both plasma cholesterol and triacylglycerol concentrations," *American Journal of Clinical Nutrition* 70, no. 6 (December 1999): 1009–15.
10. Kimberly Connor, "It's Nuts, but Keep the Fat," *Medscape Health,* 2000.
11. Denise Mann, "Taking Fish Oil Supplements a Gamble: Study," *Medscape Health,* 12 November 2001.
12. "Fiber: Still the Right Choice," *UC Berkeley Wellness Letter,* April 1999, 1–2.
13. American Institute for Cancer Research, *The Facts about Fiber,* 2001 (brochure).
14. FiberWise drink and bars available through Melaleuca, the Wellness Company, call 1-800-282-3000 or online at www.melaleuca.com.
15. National Osteoporosis Foundation, available online at www.nof.org.
16. "Not Just Milk," *UC Berkeley Wellness Letter,* January 1999, 8; USDA Nutrition Information; and product labels.
17. Revival Foods, medical grade soy, non-GMO, available from Physicians Laboratories, call 1-800-500-2055 or online at www.revivalsoy.com.
18. "Semi-Sweet Views for Your Valentine," *UC Berkeley Wellness Letter,* February 2001, 8.

19. Y. Wan et al., "Effects of cocoa powder and dark chocolate on LDL oxidative susceptibility and prostaglandin concentrations in humans," *American Journal of Nutrition* 74, no. 5 (November 2001): 596–602.
20. H. Valtin, "'Drink at least eight glasses of water a day.' Really? Is there scientific evidence for '8 x 8'?" review, *American Journal of Physiology: Regulatory, Integrative and Comparative Physiology* 283, no. 5 (November 2002): R993–1004.
21. L. E. Armstrong, "Caffeine, body fluid–electrolyte balance, and exercise performance," *International Journal of Sport Nutrition and Exercise Metabolism* 12, no. 2 (June 2002): 189–206.
22. "Green, Black, and Red: The Tea-Total Evidence," *UC Berkeley Wellness Letter,* March 2000, 1–2; "Green tea is good for you, but black tea boasts just as many benefits," *Environmental Nutrition* 25, no. 7 (July 2002): 1.
23. "Green, Black, and Red: The Tea-Total Evidence," 1; "Green tea is good for you," 4.
24. Ibid.
25. "Grounds for Celebration," in *Reader's Digest,* quoted from *Consumer Reports,* December 2001, 111–13.
26. Ibid.
27. "Filtering the News about Coffee," *UC Berkeley Wellness Letter* 17, no. 5 (February 2001): 1–2.
28. Ibid.
29. Giovannucci, "Meta-analysis of coffee consumption and risk of colorectal cancer," *American Journal of Epidemiology* 147 (1998): 1043–52.
30. P. B. Rapuri et al., "Caffeine intake increases the rate of bone loss in elderly women and interacts with vitamin D receptor genotypes," *American Journal of Clinical Nutrition* 74, no. 5 (November 2001): 694–700.
31. Data accessed 23 March 2003, online at www.coffeescience.org; "Caffeine Content—Health and Nutrition," *Time Almanac 2002,* Information Please, Learning Network, 556; "Grounds for Celebration," *Reader's Digest,* reprinted from *Consumer Reports;* "Not Just Coffee," *UC Berkeley Wellness Letter,* January 1999, 8.
32. Henry Fielding, Food Reference, available online at www.foodreference.com.

Chapter 4. Boosting Your Energy with Nutritional Supplements

1. K. M. Fairfieldx and K. M. Fairfield, "Vitamins for chronic disease prevention in adults: Clinical applications," *Journal of the American Medical Association* 287 (2002): 3127–29.

2. K. M. Fairfield and K. M. Fletcher, "Vitamins for chronic disease prevention in adults," scientific review, *Journal of the American Medical Association* 287 (2002): 3116-26.
3. "Diet and Health—Ten MegaTrends: Dietary Supplements Soar," *Nutrition Action Health Letter,* January–February 2001, 8.
4. Karen Cicero, "Is that supplement safe?" *Lifetime feature—Women's Central msn,* available online at www.womencentral.msn.com/fitnesshealth/articles.
5. "Safe Upper Limits for Common Vitamins and Minerals," Food and Nutrition Board of the Institute of Medicine, available online at www.nas.edu/iom/fnb.
6. Amanda Spake, "Natural Hazards," *U.S. News and World Report,* 12 February 2001, 48.
7. Katherine Hobson, "Danger at the Gym," *U.S. News and World Report,* 21 January 2002, 59.
8. B. J. Gurley, S. F. Gardner, and M. A. Hubbard, "Content versus label claims in ephedra-containing dietary supplements," *American Journal of Health-System Pharmacy* 57, no. 10 (15 May 2000): 963–69.
9. Rachele Kanigel, "Getting to the Root of Ginseng," *Health,* November–December 2000, 76.
10. Spake, "Natural Hazards," 43–49.
11. Michael K. Ang-Lee, Jonathan Moss, and Chun-Su Yuan, "Herbal medicines and perioperative care," *Journal of the American Medical Association* 286 (2001): 208–16.
12. J. Y. Reginster et al., "Long-term effects of glucosamine sulphate on osteoarthritis progression: A randomized, placebo-controlled clinical trial," *Lancet* 357, no. 9252 (27 January 2001): 251–56.
13. M. C. Hochberg, "What a difference a year makes: Reflections on the ACR recommendations for the medical management of osteoarthritis," review *Current Rheumatology Reports* 3, no. 6 (December 2001): 473–78.

Chapter 5. Weight-Loss Strategies That Are Wise and Energize

1. A. H. Mokdad et al., "The continuing epidemics of obesity and diabetes in the United States," *Journal of the American Medical Association* 286 (12 September 2001): 1195–1200.
2. Humphrey Taylor, "The Harris Poll #11, March 6, 2002: The Obesity Epidemic is Getting Even Worse," Harris Interactive Website, available online at www.harrisinteractive.com/harris_poll/index.asp?PID=288, accessed 24 March 2003.

3. Hallie Levine, "Health and Fitness Lies We Hate to Expose," *Glamour,* January 2000, 125.
4. National Institutes of Health, *Aim for a Healthy Weight,* calculates BMI, offers menu planner, discusses risks of obesity, available online at www.nhlbi.nih.gov/health/public/heart/obesity/lose_wt/risk.htm, accessed 24 March 2003.
5. James O. Hill, "Four Behaviors Identified That Can Spell Success in Maintaining Weight Loss," *American Medical Association,* media briefing, 12 July 2001.
6. "Meal Consumption Behavior," National Restaurant Association.
7. Adelle Davis (1904–74), "Food Reference," available online at www.foodreference.com.
8. J. M. Ashley et al., "Meal replacements in weight intervention," *Obesity Research* 9, no. 4 supplement, (November 2001): 312S–20S.
9. H. H. Ditschuneit and M. Flechtner-Mors, "Value of structured meals for weight management: Risk factors and long-term weight maintenance," *Obesity Research* 9, no. 4 supplement, (November 2001): 284S–89S.
10. J. W. Anderson et al., "Long-term weight-loss maintenance: A meta-analysis of U.S. studies," *American Journal of Clinical Nutrition* 74, no. 5 (November 2001): 579–84.
11. R. R. Wing and R. W. Jeffery, "Food provision as a strategy to promote weight loss," *Obesity Research* 9, no. 4 supplement (November 2001): 271S–75S.
12. *Lose It for Life,* call 1-800-NEW-LIFE or online at www.loseitforlife.com, *Thin Within,* call 1-877-729-8932 or online at www.thinwithinonline.com; *3D Christian Diet,* call 1-800-451-5006 or online at www.3dchristiandiet.com; *Weigh Down Workshop,* call 1-888-829-7785 or online at www.weighdown workshop.com.
13. S. Heshka et al., "Two-year randomized controlled study of self-help weight loss vs. a structured commercial program," *Federation of American Societies for Experimental Biology Journal* 15, no. 4 (Experimental Biology 2001 meeting abstracts): A623.
14. *Facts about the DASH Diet,* National Heart, Lung, and Blood Institute, available online at www.nhlbi.nih.gov/health/public/heart/hbp/new_dash.pdf; DASH diet available also by phone: 301-592-8573, or by mail: NHLBI Health Information Center, P.O. Box 30105, Bethesda, MD 20824-0105.
15. "Yet Another Health Organization Criticizes High-Protein Diets," *Tufts University Health and Nutrition Letter,* December 2001, 7.

16. C. N. Boozer et al., "An herbal supplement containing Ma Huang–Guarana for weight loss: A randomized, double-blind trial," *International Journal of Obesity Related Metabolic Disorders* 25, no. 3 (March 2001): 316–24.
17. Mark Mayell, "Healthy Highs," *Natural Health,* July–August 1998, 184.
18. E. Cunningham and W. Marcason, "Is it possible to burn calories by eating grapefruit or vinegar?" *Journal of the American Dietetic Association* 101, no. 10 (October 2001): 1198.
19. S. B. Heymsfield et al., "Garcinia cambogia (hydroxycitric acid) as a potential anti-obesity agent: A randomized controlled trial," *Journal of the American Medical Association* 280, no. 18 (11 November 1998): 1596–1600.
20. Adrienne Forman, "EN Weighs in on Over-the-Counter Weight-Loss Aids," *Environmental Nutrition,* January 2002, 2.
21. K. L. Zambell et al., "Conjugated linoleic acid supplementation in humans: Effects on body composition and energy expenditure," *Lipids* 35, no. 7 (July 2000): 777–82.
22. M. H. Pittler et al., "Randomized, double-blind trial of chitosan for body weight reduction," *European Journal of Clinical Nutrition* 53, no. 5 (May 1999): 379–81.
23. J. Umoren and C. Kies, "Commercial soybean starch blocker consumption: Impact on weight gain and on copper, lead, and zinc status of rats," *Plant Foods for Human Nutrition* 42, no. 2 (April 1992): 135–42.

Chapter 6. Exercise—A Necessary Key to the Energy You Need

1. A. H. Mokdad et al., "The continuing epidemics of obesity and diabetes in the United States," *Journal of the American Medical Association* 286 (12 September 2001): 1195–1200.
2. Daryn Eller, "Weight Gain Linked to Stress," *MSN Health,* rev. by Dr. Craig H. Kliger, available online at content.health.msn.com, accessed 30 October 2000.
3. Ibid.
4. Ibid., 48.
5. Elizabeth Trindade and Victoria Shaw, *Strollercize: The Workout for New Mothers* (New York: Three Rivers, 2001).
6. Kevin Makely, *Top Ten Fitness Fumbles,* TODAY/MSNBC.com, available online at www.msnbc.com/news/793070.asp, accessed 13 August 2002.
7. Ibid.
8. Ibid.

9. F. J. Schell, B. Allolio, and O. W. Schonecke, "Physiological and psychological effects of Hatha-Yoga exercise in healthy women," *International Journal of Psychosomatics* 41, no. 1–4 (1994): 46–52; J. J. Miller, K. Fletcher, and J. Kabat-Zinn, "Three-year follow-up and clinical implications of a mindfulness meditation-based stress reduction intervention in the treatment of anxiety disorders," *General Hospital Psychiatry* 17, no. 3 (May 1995): 192–200.
10. A. Damodaran et al., "Therapeutic potential of yoga practices in modifying cardiovascular risk profile in middle-aged men and women," *Journal of the Association of Physicians of India* 50, no. 5 (May 2002): 633–40.
11. M. Garfinkel and H. R. Schumacher Jr., "Yoga," *Rheumatic Diseases Clinics of North America* 26 no. 1 (February 2000): 125–32.
12. N. Yardi, "Yoga for control of epilepsy," *Seizure* 10, no. 1 (January 2001): 7–12.
13. A. D. Khasky and J. C. Smith, "Stress, relaxation states, and creativity," *Perceptual and Motor Skills* 88, no. 2 (April 1999): 409–16.
14. Kevin Makely, *Top Ten Fitness Fumbles.*

Chapter 7. Pick the Doctors That Are Right for You

1. Talmadge Carter, D.D.S., personal interview, 15 August 2002.

Chapter 8. Inherited Disease Risks and Screening Tests

1. Society for Women's Research, *The Leading Causes of Death for American Women,* accessed 23 March 2003, online at www.womenshealth.org.
2. E. G. Giardina, "Heart disease in women," *International Journal of Fertility and Women's Medicine* 45, no. 6 (November–December 2000): 350–57.
3. American Heart Association, *2002 Heart and Stroke Statistical Update* (Dallas: American Heart Association).
4. Nieca Goldberg, "Women Are Not Small Men," *Women's Day,* 19 February 2002, 91–98.
5. "The Wellness Guide to Preventative Care," *UC Berkeley Wellness Letter,* November 2001, 4–5.
6. American Stroke Association, accessed 24 March 2003, online at www.strokeassociation.org.
7. American Cancer Society, *Cancer Facts and Figures 2002* (Atlanta: American Cancer Society, 2002), accessed 24 March 2003, online at www.cancer.org.
8. Ibid.

9. Claudia Basquet, "Cancer and Women," excerpt from the *American Medical Women's Association Women's Complete Healthbook*, eds. Roselyn Payne Epps and Susan Cobb Stewart (Princeton, N.J.: Philip Lief Group, 1995).
10. American Cancer Society, *Cancer Facts and Figures 2002,* accessed 24 March 2003, online at www.cancer.org/downloads/STT/CFF2002.pdf.
11. American Cancer Society, *Cancer Prevention and Early Detection Facts and Figures 2002,* accessed 24 March 2003, online at www.cancer.org/downloads/STT/CPED2002.pdf.
12. *Cancer Facts and Figures 2002.*

Chapter 9. Skin Care That Makes a Difference

1. M. Huncharek and B. Kupelnick, "Use of topical sunscreens and the risk of malignant melanoma: A meta-analysis of 9067 patients from 11 case-control studies," *American Journal of Public Health* 92, no. 7 (July 2002): 1173–77.
2. Solumbria head-to-toe sun protection products, Sun Precaution Company, call 1-800-882-7860 or online at www.solumbria.com.
3. "10 rules to save your skin," *UC Berkeley Wellness Letter* 14, no. 9 (June 1998).
4. W. Stahl et al., "Carotenoids and carotenoids plus vitamin E protect against ultraviolet light-induced erythema in humans," *American Journal of Clinical Nutrition* 71, no. 3 (March 2000): 795–98.
5. *Cancer Facts and Figures 2002* and *Cancer Prevention and Early Detection Facts and Figures 2002.*
6. *Skin Cancer,* American Academy of Dermatology, accessed 24 March 2003, online at www.skincarephysicians.com/agingskinnet/Cancers.html.
7. Skincare resources include the American Academy of Dermotology (AAD), call 1-888-462-DERM or online at www.aad.org; Aging Skin Net, online at www.skincarephysicians.com/agingskinnet/.
8. OBAGI skin care information online at www.obagi.com.

Chapter 10. Physical Injury—An Occupational Hazard for Moms

1. "Table 2. Live births by age of mother, live-birth order, and race of mother: United States 2000," *National Vital Statistics Report* 50, no. 512 (February 2002).
2. Steven Copp, M.D., head of Division of Orthopedics at Scripps Clinic of San Diego, personal interview, 13 August 2002.
3. M. Quittan, "Management of back pain" review, *Disability and Rehabilitation* 24, no. 8 (20 May 2002): 423–34.

4. M. J. Verhoef, S. A. Page, and S. C. Waddell, "The Chiropractic Outcome study: Pain, functional ability and satisfaction with care," *Journal of Manipulative and Physiological Therapeutics* 20, no. 4 (May 1997): 235–40.
5. G. McMorland and E. Suter, "Chiropractic management of mechanical neck and low-back pain: A retrospective, outcome-based analysis," *Journal of Manipulative and Physiological Therapeutics* 23, no. 5 (June 2000): 307–11; L. F. Vernon, "Spinal manipulation as a valid treatment for low back pain" review, *Delaware Medical Journal* 68, no. 3 (March 1996): 175–78.
6. *A Patient's Guide to DeQuervain's Tenosynovitis,* Medical MultiMEDIA Group, available online at www.medicalmultimediagroup.com/pated/ctd/dqt/dgt.html, accessed 24 March 2003.
7. C. L. Blum, "Chiropractic and Pilates therapy for the treatment of adult scoliosis," *Journal of Manipulative and Physiological Therapeutics* 25, no. 4 (May 2002): E3.

Chapter 11. Frequent Viral Illnesses—Another Occupational Hazard for Moms

1. S. J. Sperber, "The common cold," *Infections in Medicine* 11 (1994): 235–42.
2. J. M. Gwaltney and J. O. Hendley, "Transmission of experimental rhinovirus infection by contaminated surfaces," *American Journal of Epidemiology* 116 (1982): 828–33; S. A. Sattar et al., "Chemical disinfection to interrupt the transfer of Rhinovirus type 14 from environmental surfaces to hands," *Applied and Environmental Microbiology* 59 (1993): 1579–85.
3. S. E. Reed, "An investigation on the possible transmission of rhinovirus colds through indirect contact. *Journal of Hygiene* 75 (London: 1975): 249–58.
4. Liz Vaccariello of *Fitness* magazine quoted on *OPRAH Show,* 7 June 2001 episode: "Health Mistakes Smart Women Make."
5. National Institute of Allergy and Infectious Diseases of the National Institutes of Health, "Fact Sheet: The Common Cold," available online at www.niaid.nih.gov/factsheets/cold.htm, accessed 24 March 2003; R. Eccles, "Spread of the Common Cold and Influenza," news archive from Common Cold Centre, Cardiff School of Biosciences, Cardiff University, UK, available online at www.ifh-homehygiene.org/2newspage/2new05.htm, accessed 24 March 2003.
6. B. O. Rennard et al., "Chicken soup inhibits neutrophil chemotaxis in vitro," *Ches* 118, no. 4 (October 2000): 1150–57.
7. "Fact Sheet: The Common Cold."

8. R. M. Brinkeborn et al, "Echinaforce and other Echinacea fresh plant preparations in the treatment of the common cold," *Phytomedicine* 6, no. 1 (March 1999): 1–5.
9. Skye Lininger et al., "Astragalus," in *The Natural Pharmacy* (Rocklin, Calif.: Prima, 1998), 234.
10. D. T. Chu, W. L. Wong, and G. M. Mavligit, "Immunotherapy with Chinese medicinal herbs. II. Reversal of cyclophosphamide-induced immune suppression by administration of fractionated Astragalus membranaceus in vivo," *Journal of Clinical & Laboratory Immunology* 25, no. 3 (March 1988): 125–29.
11. Randy W. Brown, "Final Report for Protocol KML001—Airborne Clinical Trial," 12 November 2002. GNG Pharmaceutical Services, Inc. Sugarloaf, Florida, call 305-745-1472.
12. A. S. Prasad et al., "Duration of symptoms and plasma cytokine levels in patients with the common cold treated with zinc acetate," *Annals of Internal Medicine* 133 (2000): 245–52.
13. Donal O'Mathuna and Walt Larimore, "Zinc," in *Alternative Medicine: The Christian Handbook* (Grand Rapids, 2001), 462–63.
14. Z. Zakay-Rones et al., "Inhibition of several strains of influenza virus in vitro and reduction of symptoms by an elderberry extract (Sambucus nigra L.) during an outbreak of influenza B Panama," *Journal of Alternative and Complementary Medicine* 1, no. 4 (Winter 1995): 361–69.
15. V. Barak, T. Halperin, and I. Kalickman, "The effect of Sambucol, a black elderberry-based, natural product, on the production of human cytokines: I. Inflammatory cytokines," *European Cytokine Network,* 12, no. 2 (April–June 2001): 290–96.

Chapter 12. The Benefits of Wise Lifestyle Choices

1. Maggie Scarf, *Intimate Partner* (New York: Ballantine, 1996).
2. *UC Berkeley Wellness Letter,* April 2000, 8.
3. I. Kawachi et al., "A prospective study of passive smoking and coronary heart disease," *Circulation* 95 (1997): 2374–79.
4. T. Eissenberg, "Smokers' sex and the effects of tobacco cigarettes: Subject-rated and physiological measures," *Nicotine and Tobacco Research Journal* 1, no. 4 (December 1999): 317–24.
5. *M.D./Alert Tips* number 97:11. Continuing education resource available online at www.alertmarketing.com.
6. J. Manuel, "A healthy home environment?" *Environmental Health Perspective* 107, no. 7 (July 1999): A352–427.

7. Richard Barry, *Let's Stop Poisoning Our Children!* (Littleton, Colo.: R.M. Barry Publications, 1996), source of information: "Accident Facts, 1993" National Safety Council.
8. R. Das and P. D. Blanc, "Chlorine gas exposure and the lung," a review, *Toxicology and Industrial Health* 9, no. 3 (May–June 1993): 439–55.
9. J. P. Zock, M. Kogevinas, and J. Sunyer, "Asthma risk, cleaning activities and use of specific cleaning products among Spanish indoor cleaners," *Scandinavian Journal of Work, Environment, and Health* 27, no. 1 (February 2001): 76–81.
10. Barry, *Let's Stop Poisoning Our Children!*
11. Ecosense Cleaning Products, Melaleuca, Wellness Company, call 1-800-282-3000 or available online at www.melaleuca.com.
12. Miracle Clean Products by Joy Mangano, order through Home Shopping Network, call 1-800-284-3100 or available online at www.hsn.com.
13. Simple Green, available in retail stores, for store location, call 1-800-228-0709 or available online at www.simplegreen.com.
14. M. C. Marbury, G. Maldonado, and L. Waller, "The indoor air and children's health study: Methods and incidence rates," *Epidemiology* 7, no. 2 (March 1996): 166–74.

Chapter 13. Libido, Libido . . . Where's My Libido?

1. Kegel Exercises.com, available online at www.kegelexercises.com/kegel_exercises/kegel_exercises.html, accessed 24 March 2003.

Chapter 14. Safe Birth Control

1. Gene Rudd, M.D., associate executive director Christian Medical and Dental Associations (22 August 2002), unpublished statement.
2. Review article by Joseph Spinnato, *American Journal of Obstetrics and Gynecology* 176 (1997): 503–6.
3. Sources: Joe McIlhaney Jr. and Susan Nethery, "Chapter 12: Birth Control—Temporary and Permanent," *1001 Health-Care Questions Women Ask,* 3rd ed. (Grand Rapids: Baker, 1998), 485–513; FDA Office of Public Affairs, U.S. Food and Drug Administration, *Birth Control Guide,* updated 12 August 2002, available online at www.fda.gov/fdac/features/1997/babytabl.html#a; Tamar Nordenberg, "Protecting against Unintended Pregnancy: A Guide to Contraceptive Choices," *U.S. Food and Drug Administration FDA Consumer Magazine,* revised June 2000, available online at www.fda.gov/fdac/features/1997/397_baby.html; *Thinking about Birth Control,* McKinley Health

Center, University of Illinois at Urbana-Champaign website, www.mckinley.uiuc.edu/health-info/sexual/birthcon/thnk-bc.html; *Some Options for Birth Control,* Plainsense.com, available online at www.plainsense.com/Health/Womens/cntrcptn.htm; Colleen McNally, M.D., ob-gyn, vice-chief for Ob-Gyn Department at Sharp Memorial Hospital, San Diego, chairman of Bioethics Department for San Diego Sharp Hospitals, member of North American Menopausal Society, June 2002, personal interview.

4. McIlhaney and Nethery, "Birth Control—Temporary and Permanent," 485–513.

Chapter 15. When Getting Pregnant Again Isn't So Easy

1. Study by Wilcox et al., *New England Journal of Medicine* 331 (1995): 1517–21; quoted in Joe McIlhaney Jr. and Susan Nethery, "The initial fertility exam," *1001 Health-Care Questions Women Ask,* 3rd ed. (Grand Rapids: Baker, 1998), 437.
2. Jennifer Warner, "Many Can Wait for Fertility Treatment—Most couples conceive naturally within two years," WebMD, information from study by David Duncan, M.D., National Institute of Environmental Health Sciences in North Carolina; presented his findings July 2002 at conference of European Society of Human Reproduction and Embryology.
3. M. Sara Rosenthal, "Basal Body Temperature Chart (Symptothermal Method)," *The Fertility Sourcebook* (Columbus, Ohio: McGraw-Hill RGA, 1998), available online at webmd.lycos.com/content/article/1680.51216, accessed 24 March 2003.
4. "Pregnancy—Identifying fertile days," Medline Plus Health Information / National Institutes of Health, updated 12 June 2001, available online at www.nlm.nih.gov/medlineplus/ency/article/007015.htm.
5. Warner, "Many Can Wait."
6. Pregnancy odds each month data from Reproductive Medicine Associates of New Jersey, in Nancy Gibbs, "Making Time for a Baby," *TIME,* 15 April 2002, 50–54.
7. Ibid., 51.
8. J. K. Wilson and E. J. Kopitzke, "Stress and Infertility," *Current Women's Health Rep* 2, no. 3 (June 2002): 194–99.
9. Timothy McCall, "Get a healthier, frazzle-free life," *Redbook,* September 2001, 28.

10. J. Wright et al., "Psychosocial distress and infertility: A review of controlled research," *International Journal of Fertility* 34, no. 2 (March–April 1989): 126–42.
11. Maria Essig, "Infertility Testing," *Medical Encyclopedia,* 30 May 2000.
12. American Society of Reproductive Medicine, "What is in vitro fertilization?" available online at www.asrm.org/Patients/faqs.html, accessed 24 March 2003.
13. Reproductive Science Center of San Francisco, "Assisted Reproductive Technologies," available online at www.rscbayarea.com/services/artindex.html, accessed 24 March 2003.
14. About.com, "Infertility Treatment Drugs," available online at www.infertility.about.com/library/ifctr/bldrugs.htm, accessed 24 March 2003.
15. Advanced Reproductive Care, "Infertility Information, Treatments—GIFT," available online at www.arcfertility.com/infertility/infertility_treatments.html, accessed 24 March 2003.
16. The following are good resources for infertility: Support group, RESOLVE: National Infertility Association, available online at www.resolve.org or call 617-623-0744; American Infertility Association, available online at www.americaninfertility.org or call 718-621-5083; and American Society for Reproductive Medicine, available online at www.asrm.org or call 205-978-5000.
17. American Society for Reproductive Medicine, "ASRM: State Insurance Laws," available online at www.asrm.org/Patients/insur.html, accessed 24 March 2003.

Chapter 16. Those Fluctuating Hormones—From PMS to Perimenopause

1. "How is PMDD Different from Premenstrual Syndrome (PMS)?" *Premenstrual Dysphoric Disorder (PMDD)* in Medem Medical Library with American Psychiatric Association (2001), available online at www.medem.com, accessed 24 March 2003.
2. S. Thys-Jacobs et al., "Calcium carbonate and the premenstrual syndrome: Effects on premenstrual and menstrual symptoms," *American Journal of Obstetrics and Gynecology* 179 (1998): 444–52.
3. A. F. Walker et al., "Magnesium supplementation alleviates premenstrual symptoms of fluid retention," *Journal of Women's Health* 7 (1998): 1157–65; F. Facchinetti et al., "Oral magnesium successfully relieves premenstrual mood changes," *Obstetrics and Gynecology* 78 (1991) 177–81; F. Facchinetti et al., "Magnesium prophylaxis of menstrual migraine: Effects on intracellular magnesium," *Headache* 31 (1991): 298–301.

4. Adrianne Bendich, "The potential for dietary supplements to reduce premenstrual syndrome (PMS) symptoms," *Journal of the American College of Nutrition* 19, no. 1 (2000): 3–12.
5. *Appendix of the Diagnostic and Statistical Manual of Mental Disorders,* 4th ed. (Washington, D.C.: American Psychiatric Association, 1994).
6. North American Menopause Society, "Basic facts about menopause," available online at www.menopause.org/aboutm/facts.html, accessed 7 November 2000.
7. J. Guthrie et al., "Hot flashes, menstrual status, and hormone levels in a population-based sample of midlife women," *Obstetrics and Gynecology* 88 (1996): 437–42.
8. Amanda Spake, "Hormones on Trial," *U.S. News and World Report,* 21 January 2002, 54.
9. Statement by Colleen McNally, M.D., regarding hormone replacement therapy, 29 July 2002.
10. Andrew Weil, "Rethinking Hormone Therapy," *Dr. Andrew Weil's Self Healing Newsletter* (Watertown, Mass.: Thorne Communications, September 2002), 1.
11. L. J. Lu, J. A. Tice, and F. L. Bellino, "Phytoestrogens and healthy aging: Gaps in knowledge. A workshop report," *Menopause* 8, no. 3 (May–June 2001): 157–70.
12. K. Elkind-Hirsch, "Effect of dietary phytoestrogens on hot flashes: Can soy-based proteins substitute for traditional estrogen replacement therapy?" *Menopause* 8, no. 3 (May–June 2001): 154–56.
13. Revival non-GMO, not chemically processed, soy foods from Physicians Laboratory, available online at www.revivalsoy.com or call 1-800-500-2055.
14. "Herbal medicine: Black Cohosh: The woman's herb?" *Harvard Women's Health Watch* 7, no. 8 (April 2000): 6.
15. "Black Cohosh: Was Lydia E. Pinkham on to Something?" *UC Berkeley Wellness Letter,* February 2001, 5.
16. Adriane Fugh-Berman and Fredi Kronenberg, "Red clover (Trifolium pratense) for menopausal women: Current state of knowledge," *Menopause* 8 (2001): 333–37.
17. J. D. Hirata et al. "Does dong quai have estrogenic effects in postmenopausal women? A double-blind, placebo-controlled trial," *Fertility and Sterility* 68, no. 6 (December 1997): 981–86.

18. Elizabeth Ward, "Health Concerns at Menopause: HRT vs. Natural Remedies for Relief," *Environmental Nutrition,* January 2000, 4.

Chapter 17. Mom's Mental Health—Feeling Blue Rather Than Tickled Pink

1. National Institute of Mental Health, available online at www.nimh.nih.gov/publicat/numbers.cfm, accessed 24 March 2003.
2. Katherine L. Wisner, Barbara L. Parry, and Catherine M. Piontek, "Postpartum Depression," *New England Journal of Medicine* 347, no. 3 (18 July 2002): 194–99.
3. Paul Meier, M.D. and panel, "Understanding Mental Illness I–II," radio broadcast on Focus on the Family, 29 July 2002, available on cassette #CT452 or online at www.family.org or call 1-800-A-FAMILY (1-800-232-6459).
4. Paul Meier, Stephen Arterburn, and Frank Minirth, *Mood Swings* (Nashville: Nelson, 2000).
5. Minirth-Meier New Life Clinics, located in sixteen states, available online at www.newlife.com/Meier/Clinics/meier_clinics.htm or call 1-800-NEW-LIFE (1-800-639-5433).
6. M. Bloch et al., "Effects of gonadal steroids in women with a history of postpartum depression," *American Journal of Psychiatry* 157 (2000): 924–30.
7. C. T. Beck, "Predictors of postpartum depression: An update (meta-analysis)," *Nursing Research* 50, no. 5 (2001): 275–85.
8. K. L. Wisner and Z. N. Stowe, "Psychobiology of postpartum mood disorders," *Seminars in Reproductive Endocrinology* 15 (1997): 77–89.
9. K. L. Wisner, K. S. Peindl, and B. H. Hanusa, "Symptomatology of affective and psychotic illnesses related to childbearing," *Journal of Affective Disorders* 30 (1994): 77–87; B. L. Parry and J. Hamilton, "Postpartum Psychiatric Syndromes," in *The Art of Psychopharmacology,* eds. S. C. Risch and D. S. Janowsky (New York: Guilford, 1992).
10. F. Dimeo et al., "Benefits from aerobic exercise in patients with major depression: A pilot study," *British Journal of Sports Medicine* 35, no. 2 (April 2001): 114–17.
11. H. G. Koenig, "Psychoneurimmunology and the faith factor," *Journal of Gender Specific Medicine* 3, no. 5 (July–August 2000): 37–44.
12. S. W. Lazar et al., "Functional brain mapping of the relaxation response and meditation," *Neuroreport* 11, no. 7 (2000): 1581–85.
13. H. Hiscock and M. Wake, "Infant sleep problems and postnatal depression: A community-based study," *Pediatrics* 107, no. 6 (June 2001): 1317–22.

14. R. Shelton et al., "Effectiveness of St. John's wort in major depression, a randomized controlled trial," *Journal of the American Medical Association* 285 (18 April 2001): 1978–86.
15. "Don't Take the Herb Kava," *UC Berkeley Wellness Letter,* March 2002, 8.

Acknowledgments

I battled with Ménière's disease and health issues throughout the writing of this book. Without the support of many important people in my life, this book would not exist.

To my husband, Gary Chun, M.D., son, Robert Chun, and Theo: Thank you for every level of support you provided and your unconditional love. From doing laundry, getting take-out meals, understanding when I needed to work instead of play, to encouraging me when the task seemed impossible; your actions and love sustained me. Robert, thank you for frequently asking, "How are you doing, Mom?" I am so grateful you are my family.

To Chip (Jerry) MacGregor, my agent extraordinaire: Thank you for recommending me for this project, and for your amazing support every step of the way. You always go the extra mile—I hope to work with you for decades to come. Thank you also to Alice Crider and Andrea Christian, Chip's assistants, for your faithful support, friendship, and prayers. Thank you, Alive Communications; it is a privilege to be one of your authors. Marie Prys, thank you for your superb editing. Megan Gorris, thank you for administrative expertise.

To Zondervan: Thank you for publishing this book. Special thanks to Executive Editor Sandy Vander Zicht, who is not only a gifted editor but also a caring and supportive leader.

To Zondervan's Associate Editor Angela Scheff, Cindy Hays Lambert, Holli Leegwater, Angela Rottier, Cindy Wilcox, and Sue Brower in marketing, and all the others behind the scenes: You all have worked so hard to make this the best book possible. I appreciate each of you!

To MOPS International: Thank you for asking me to partner with you to provide this resource for moms. It is a joy to work with each of you. Special thanks to MOPS editor Beth Lagerborg. You are the perfect combination of editor, counselor, and supportive girlfriend.

To CLASServices: Thank you for excellent training, superb support, and for introducing me to my agent, Chip MacGregor. To the San Diego Christian Writers Guild: Thank you for your encouragement and professional support.

To the experts who shared their wisdom: Talmadge Carter, D.D.S., Steven Copp, M.D., Bill Dascombe, M.D., Nancy Deason, MFCC, Zoe Draelos, M.D., Marita Littauer, Colleen McNally, M.D., Anthony Oro, M.D., Gene Rudd, M.D., Tom Syta, and Aaron Tabor, M.D. Your expertise is what makes this book a wonderful resource. Thank you also to Patricia Buckley and Joanne Puszykowski, who shared their expertise as mothers.

To my mom, Joyce Bloemer: Thank you for being such an admirable mom, and *my* mom. You are a tough act to follow—but I'm trying! Ray Bloemer, thank you for your support and encouragement. I'm glad you are one of the family.

To my dad, Tal Carter and his bride, Cala Carter: Thank you both for your love and support.

To Maybelle Whang, my Chinese mother: Thank you for your encouragement and for sponsoring our family reunion each year.

To Grandma Mazie Cooper and cousin Dana Crouch: Thank you for your abundant prayers, encouragement, and support.

To Karen Lew, my "little sister": You are such a gifted encourager! Thank you for the countless ways you spur me on to write well and live well.

To Peggy Ngubo: Thank you for being the friend that I can always call for help—whether it be to take me to the doctor or post office, or to sit with me and pray. May God bless you for your faithfulness!

To Michele Bluhm (and Wolfgang) who faithfully bless us with gourmet meals: Thank you for your generosity and support.

To the many friends from Solana Beach Presbyterian church: Thank you for your support and prayers.

To Carol Slomka, Michelle Hooten, Barbara Shooter, and Mandy Forssman: Thank you for being such special friends, chauffeurs, counselors, and prayer partners. You've eased my load and warmed my heart more times than you know.

To the Moms in Touch prayer group at the Evans School, Deborah Fabian (my coleader), Jill Champion, Traci Espeseth, Mandy Forssman, Rhonda Gallegos, Deborah Greenspan, Michelle Hooten, Diane LaDouce, Allison Lane, Susan Littlejohn, Ioana Partovi, Gloria Patino, Rosa Robertson, Gretchen Sargeant, Barbara Shooter, and Carol Slomka: Thank you for your prayer support! You are phenomenal, faithful mothers.

To Gale Baer and Marianne Augustine: Thank you for the countless ways you have supported our family. I learn more about grace and generosity the longer I know you. Thank you also to the rest of the staff of the Evans School for your encouragement and investment in our son, Robert.

To Jim and Carole Leavengood, Bobby Simmons, Rick Meads, Ralph Johnson, Annette and Ron Allen, Patricia and Mike Buckley, Allen and Belva Warkentin, and Roylee York: Thank you for your friendship and prayer support.

To Edie Warkentin, Terri Huber, and Glenn Thomson: Thank you for being such caring friends. Thank you to the many other family friends who have encouraged and cared.

To Sheryl and Paul Russell and those in Christian Community Theater: Thank you for your prayers and support throughout my illness.

To Dee Tarango (an inspiring Ménière's disease survivor): Thank you for pouring out your knowledge and encouragement when I became ill.

To Anna Berquist, Martha Stalker, my other office staff, and the pediatricians who have been my partners, Jeffrey Selzer, M.D., Arlene Wong, M.D., Stuart Cohen, M.D., Shawn Bissonnette, M.D.: Thank you for all your support and for all you have taught me through the years.

To the nurses of Scripps Hospital Labor and Delivery and Postpartum units, Ken Curzon (my faithful friend), and our lunch bunch: Thank you for being such important people in my professional life.

Special thanks to my friend, Phil Paleologas of "American Breakfast with Phil Paleologas" national radio show: Your support for my writing means more than I can say. Thank you for your friendship and your support on-air and off.

The greatest thanks of all goes to my heavenly father who makes all things possible, made every page of this book possible, and surprises me constantly with his grace and provision. To God be the glory!

Index

The MOPS Story

MOPS stands for Mothers of Preschoolers, a program designed to encourage mothers with children under school age through relationships and resources. These women come from different backgrounds and lifestyles, yet have similar needs and a shared desire to be the best mothers they can be!

A MOPS group provides a caring, accepting atmosphere for today's mother of preschoolers. Here she has an opportunity to share concerns, explore areas of creativity, and hear instruction that equips her for the responsibilities of family and community. The MOPS group also includes MOPPETS, a loving, learning experience for children.

Approximately 2,700 groups meet in churches throughout the United States, Canada, and 19 other countries, to meet the needs of more than 100,000 women. Many more mothers are encouraged by MOPS resources, including *MOMSense* radio and magazine, MOPS' web site, and publications such as this book.

Find out how MOPS International can help you become part of MOPS ♥to♥ Mom Connection.

MOPS International

2370 South Trenton Way

Denver, CO 80231-3822

Phone 1-800-929-1287 or 303-733-5353

E-mail: Info@MOPS.org

Web site: http://www.MOPS.org

To learn how to start a MOPS group, call 1-800-910-MOPS.

For MOPS products call The MOPShop 1-800-545-4040.

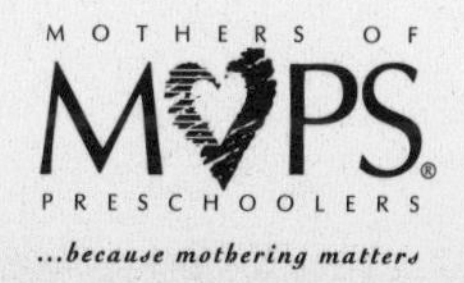

We want to hear from you. Please send your comments about this book to us in care of zreview@zondervan.com. Thank you.

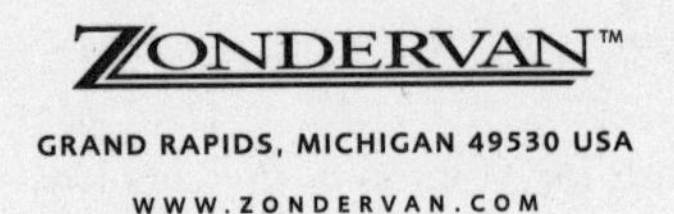

GRAND RAPIDS, MICHIGAN 49530 USA

WWW.ZONDERVAN.COM